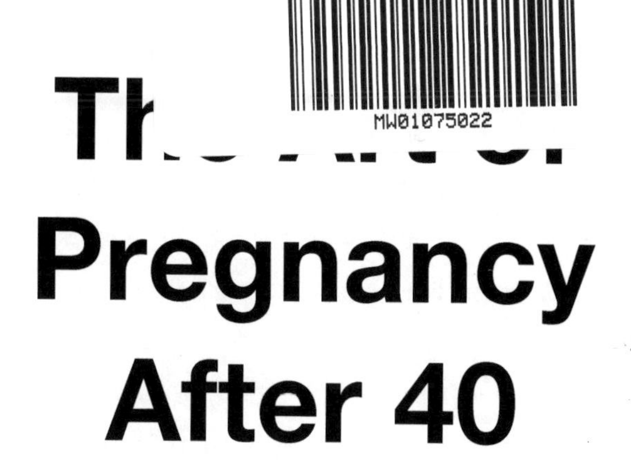

Pregnancy After 40

A Personal Journey, Medical Standards, Myths, and the Latest Research

Expanded and Updated Edition

Katka Konecna-Rivera

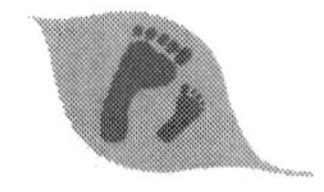

Living Green with Baby

This book is written as a source of information only, and should not be considered as a substitute for the advice, decisions, or judgment of qualified health professionals. All efforts have been made to ensure the accuracy of the information contained in this book as of the date published. The author and the publisher expressly disclaim responsibility for any adverse affects arising from the use or application of the information contained herein.

Second Edition with expanded and updated information published in January 2017.

ISBN-13: 978-1530351541

ISBN-10: 1530351545

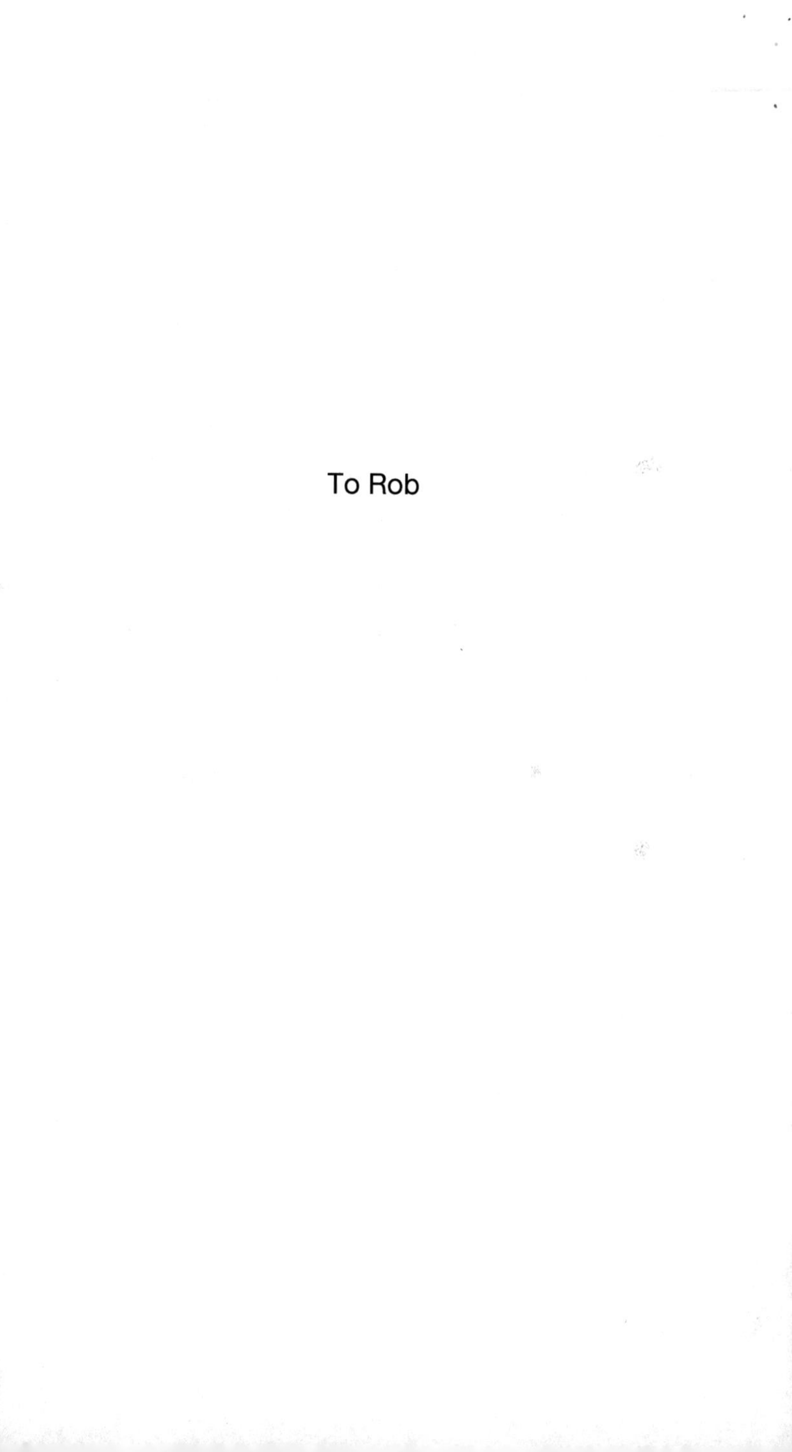
To Rob

Contents

Introduction

As we say in Czech,

"There is no cure for aging."

Alright, here comes the BIG 40. You've worked hard, played hard, and before you realize it, you are officially *old*.

It seems like a lifetime away when I was 20. Yet that milestone came in a blink of an eye. I remember thinking about the year 2000 as a distant star in another universe; and when it actually came, it was nothing but another number. I felt the same way about turning 40 and did not even celebrate it as anything special. Yet turning forty might not feel the same to others. To some people, it might be a benchmark to classify a woman as officially *old*. What does that mean anyway? It means you shouldn't look at younger men; otherwise you might be classified as a "cougar," you shouldn't dress sexy, you shouldn't act funny, you shouldn't drink too much, you shouldn't do this or that...the list goes on.

On the other hand, more and more women

today delay getting married and having babies until their late 30s or 40s for both professional and personal reasons. I often hear: “Forty is the new 30; 50 is the new 40.” In my opinion, it’s all relative. Every woman can feel differently about family, career, relationship, or life in general, and it’s her right to choose any path she’s comfortable with.

Then there is the perception of older people, who see women in their 40s as still very young, with about a half of their lifetime ahead of them. Since they already know what comes after 40, their perspective is somehow very comforting.

However, society and the media often paint a different picture, especially in some professions and social circles. The constant pressure of looking “young” and keeping up with the younger peers have forced many women to undergo unnecessary procedures, lifestyle changes and even surgeries, which often have a negative impact on their physical and mental health.

So what are you allowed to do when you reach that “critical” point? I don’t think there is a universal answer to this question. Each woman is unique in her own way and might have her personal view on her life and where she stands when she reaches 40. Therefore, all I would say is: “Take what others say with a grain of salt; this is your own life, and only you can live it. Instead, listen to your instincts, spend some quality time with and for yourself only, and focus on your well-being, both physical and emotional.“

Chapter 1: Baby After 40

As we say in Czech,

"Don't get old until you get smart."

As much as I'm trying to understand the beauty of pregnancy, I have to admit that there wasn't much I can say I really enjoyed about being pregnant. Actually, maybe I should confess that I really hated it, especially the second time around. I've met women who raved about loving being pregnant, but I personally don't get it. A friend of mine recently told me that she would really like to have another child and a sibling for her 5-year-old daughter, but the idea of going through yet another nightmarish pregnancy is making her very hesitant. "If somebody handed me a newborn today, I would be totally happy and a great mom to both kiddos, but dealing with 9 months of suffering like the last time, plus the additional stress from all the genetic testing now that I'm over 35, is really making me shiver." I know exactly what she means, and if I ever have another child, I'm going to close down the shop right after.

When I found out I was pregnant for the first

time at the age of 36, it was like "whaaat"?! I had just gotten off my birth control for certain health reasons, and my long-time gynecologist (and friend) assured me that at my age I wouldn't have to worry about getting pregnant for at least 6 months. So I didn't. And two months later I was pregnant. That freaked me out at first. Then I thought about my life and concluded that I had pretty much already "done everything I wanted to do in my life," and maybe it was time for another chapter, which included parenting.

My first pregnancy was surprisingly easy; I was fit and had a pretty healthy lifestyle, so the only adjustments and sacrifices I had to make included coffee, alcohol, sushi, scuba diving, surfing, and few other "goodies." Everything else was pretty much just like before.

But now, 4 years later, things might be a little different. This time I'm thinking about planned pregnancy, and I bet it won't be as smooth as before. From my humble, yet deep research, it appears as though the chances for a natural and healthy pregnancy after 40 are pretty slim, but not impossible.

And why have I decided to have another child?

Quite frankly, after my first baby I wasn't sure I could handle another. Not that my boy was a difficult baby, but I was quite worn out. But later on, seeing my boy's buddies playing with their siblings, I felt that maybe it would be good for him to have a sibling too, and maybe it would be good for us (me and my husband) to have a second child, so we are not too uptight about him.

As I opened up about writing this book to some of my girlfriends, I learned that miscarriages and fertility problems are much more common than I have imagined—even among women who are in their 20s or early 30s.

Here are some of the stats on pregnancy after 40, according to the American Society for Reproductive Medicine (ASRM) and courtesy of BabyCenter:

- *About 50% of women have fertility problems*
- *There is a 5% chance of getting pregnant in any single ovulation cycle*
- *A chance of conceiving within a year of beginning to try is about 40–50% (compared to a woman in her mid-30s, who has a 75% chance)*

- *From 40–44, the miscarriage rate is 35%, and it rises to over 50% from 45 and older (compared to 10% at age 20 and 12% at 30)*
- *The risk of pregnancy complications, such as high blood pressure and diabetes, is twice as high as for a woman in her 20s.*

Although it's good to know these facts, I wouldn't stress over them. All right, I'm having one of my last drinks (a glass of Shiraz) right now, since I need to call it quits pretty soon. What else have I missed?

Since scientists never sleep, for better or worse, there are constantly new studies coming out with new (and sometimes conflicting) findings. For example, results from a 2014 study published in the *International Journal of Epidemiology*[1] suggest that the risk of giving birth to a child with an autism spectrum disorder is much higher for women after age 30 and the same goes for older men fathering a child. While other new studies have more encouraging findings. New research from Birkbeck University published in the *European Journal of Developmental Psychology*[2] indicates that older

[1] Parental age and the risk of autism spectrum disorders

[2] The parenting of preschool children by older mothers in the United Kingdom

mothers (30 or over) are more likely to parent responsibly and, compared to teenage mothers, are less likely to use harsh punishments like spanking their children. Other studies[3] also show that older mothers seem to provide safer environments for their children; results show that children are 22% less likely to accidentally injure themselves and almost a third less likely to be admitted to a hospital by age 3 due to non-underlying health problems. The study also indicates that older mothers may be better suited to deal with parent-child conflict. In addition to these encouraging findings, new preliminary research[4] from Washington University in St. Louis suggests that while chromosomal defects do rise with maternal age, congenital defects[5] don't follow that same trend.

So I guess there is some hope for us older moms after all.

---

[3] The health and development of children born to older mothers in the United Kingdom

[4] Women 35 and older have a lower risk of having anatomically abnormal children

[5] A congenital defect or birth defect is a congenital abnormality, congenital anomaly, or congenital disorder— a condition existing at birth and often before birth, or that develops during the first month of life.

Chapter 2: Done with the Pill

Baby number 2 is on my mind; therefore, today is the last day before the first day. That sounds quite dramatic, I know. Today I'm taking my last birth control pill and beginning a new chapter, hopefully. And what happens next? After my next period, there will be a lot of sex on the horizon—for better or worse.

In the meantime, I need to "clean up" my act and get my old body ready for what might be coming. What does that mean, exactly? Alcohol goes first. As much as I believe that a glass of red wine every now and then wouldn't harm the future sprout, it's better to keep it clean at this age. Coffee is next. Actually, since my first pregnancy I kept it at one cup of brew a day, so if I stick to my morning routine, I should be fine. What's next? Exercise: ever since I herniated a disc in my lower back about six months ago, I have kept my regular routine in check, meaning no running, lifting, or any other stress on my lower back. I stuck to my daily yoga and core workouts, including push-ups and walking. Today I'm almost back to normal (I would say about 98%), and maybe I should start running again. Hmm, but when do I have time for running in my busy schedule? I'm not exactly a gym lover, so I guess I should talk my man into buying a treadmill. I know it sounds like an unnecessary piece of equipment, but honestly that's the only way I can see myself running 3 times a week. From what I've seen recently, there are "light" models that can be easily stored in a corner and that are pretty inexpensive too. I could include it in the "baby budget," and nobody will have an issue with that.

Chapter 3: I Want a Girl

Yes, nature can't guarantee anything but a fifty-fifty chance of conceiving a girl or a boy, and science strictly confirms it[6]. There is nothing I can do to affect that. But, according to some "natural mamas," over the course of history there has been some evidence that we can affect our preference to a certain point. I dove into my research and after reading a lot and watching many "educational" videos, I almost felt nauseous from some of the stuff I saw and heard. According to Dr. Shettles, sometimes referred to as "father of the in vitro fertilization (IVF)," the timing of the intercourse and a few other details increase the mother's chances of influencing her baby's sex. Alright, now I'm ready to give it a try. I'm fresh off the pill, so what do I have to do before my "fertile period" begins? What? No caffeine? Are you serious, Dr. Shettles! How am I going to get through my day without my morning coffee?

---

[6] Since we're talking science, in most countries male births are slightly higher than female births. Specifically, for each conception, there's about a 52% chance it will be a boy.

Here is the Shettles Theory to conceiving a girl:

- *You should have sex 2–3 days before ovulation to allow the Y-bearing sperm to die off before the egg becomes available during ovulation.*
- *Women should avoid orgasms because it makes the vagina less favorable for the X-bearing sperm that prefer the acidic environment.*
- *Avoid sexual positions that involve deep penetration.*

Alright, two cycles later, no success conceiving, so either this method is not very effective (given that we are supposed to avoid the actual ovulation day) or we are doing something wrong. Oh well, at least we are still enjoying ourselves!

My skeptical scientist husband gives me a smirk and adds, "Don't you think that if this really worked, countries like China and North Korea would have been breeding boys for their armies for decades already? Of course it doesn't work!"

Chapter 4: Twins or Other Multiples

After 35, the chance of conceiving twins or other multiples significantly increases since older women might release more than one egg during ovulation. According to a 2009 report by the Centers for Disease Control and Prevention (CDC), in the United States, about 7% of all births for women 40 and older were twins, compared to 5% of women in their late 30s and 2% of women age 24 or younger. That still doesn't sounds huge, statistically, but it's definitely another fact to think about.

My husband totally freaked me out one day when he joked about conceiving triplets after a massive ejaculation! I guess now I just have to wait and see what comes of it.

And what if, hypothetically speaking, we ended up with twins? Honestly, that's a thought that I would prefer not to focus on at all. A friend and neighbor recently had twin boys. She already has a 4-year old boy and had been trying to get pregnant for several years without success. And now she's got twins. She and her husband seem super happy—although having 3 boys in a house is something I'd rather not think about. Plus, she's like 15 years younger than me! I guess we'll go with the flow, see what happens, and deal with it as it comes.

There are stories though, that are worth sharing since they can be very inspirational to others. A new friend of mine I became very close with opened up about her very unique experience. She accidentally got pregnant in her late 40s despite contraception. When she was experiencing sudden health issues and intense pain in her abdomen, she requested medical help and went through all sorts of tests to determine the cause. She was ready for the worst, when a sonogram of her pancreas revealed that she was pregnant. Although it was a shocker to her and her family, it was a relief at the same time, since she wasn't "dying." They started preparing for the new reality of having a baby with two kids in college. Then a required genetic test indicated a super high risk of Down syndrome. She and her husband decided to continue the pregnancy anyways. A few weeks later, when driving her two kids to school, she started bleeding excessively, which was a sign of miscarriage. It wasn't a huge surprise, given her age, yet still a heartbreaking experience. Several more weeks went by and the intense pain hadn't subsided. During another doctor visit, they discovered she was originally pregnant with twins, one baby died and got flushed out of her uterus, and the other was alive. When her baby boy was born, he was well and healthy. It turned out that the baby who died had Down syndrome and nature had done its selection early.

Chapter 5: Father's Diet and Supplements Before Conception

Judging according to my own father and my husband, both educated and health-conscious men, most men really don't care about vitamins and supplements, let alone consider them important for the quality of their sperm. Yet, according to a new study led by McGill researcher Sarah Kimmins[7], the father's diet before conception may play an equally important role in the baby's health as the mother's diet does. The research focused on vitamin B9 (also called folate), which is well known to be crucial for a healthy pregnancy, has shown that folate levels of the father are just as important. The results indicate that future fathers should pay the same attention to their lifestyle and diet before conceiving a child, just like mothers do.

But if you are dealing with a stubborn man who doesn't believe in science and research, or you want to make sure he's "loaded" with the good stuff, consider

---

[7] Father's diet before conception

adding the following foods that are naturally high in folate to his diet:

- *Beans-cooked*: black-eyed peas (52% daily value (DV)), mung beans (80%), pinto beans (74%), chickpeas (71%), pink beans (71%), lima beans (68%), black beans (64%), navy beans (64%), and kidney beans (58%);
- *Lentils-cooked* (45% DV);
- *Spinach-raw* (49% DV); other dark-green leafy veggies (%DV per cup cooked): turnip greens (42%), bok choi-Chinese cabbage (17%), Savoy cabbage (17%), and collard greens (8%);
- *Asparagus-cooked* (37%);
- *Lettuce* -Cos or Romaine (37%), other lettuce veggies (%DV per cup shredded): endive (18%), butterhead (10%), salad cress (10%), chicory (8%), and arugula;
- *Avocado* (20%);
- *Broccoli-cooked* (27%);

- *Other brassica veggies* (%DV per cup cooked): Chinese broccoli (22%), broccoli raab (15%), and cauliflower (14%);
- *Mango* (11%);
- *Other tropical fruit* (%DV per fruit): pomegranate (27%), papaya (15%), guava (7%), kiwi (7%), and banana (6%);
- *Oranges* (10%);
- *Wheat bread* (21%);
- *Other breads* (%DV per slice): French bread (24%), Italian bread (14%), and wheat germ bread (8%).

Good luck!

Chapter 6: Quinine

Growing up in the Czech Republic, I was always surrounded by a lot of good beer and liquor, including an herbal liquor called *Becherovka*, nowadays famous worldwide. Becherovka has some medicinal properties, given the fact that it contains about a hundred different medicinal herbs, but its combination with tonic water and lemon makes a delicious and popular drink. In Czech it's nicknamed "BeTon" (short for Becherovka-tonic), which means concrete in English. It's been my personal favorite mixed drink ever since I could officially drink alcohol; maybe being an engineer-architect has something to do with it.

Here comes the double NO-NO if you're planning on becoming pregnant or are already there: 1. hard liquor-definitely not; 2. tonic water-better not. Why? Because tonic water contains *quinine*, a bitter-tasting, crystalline powder obtained from the bark of the cinchona tree. Although the alkaloid is used as medicine to treat malaria and nocturnal calf muscle cramps, it can pass through the placenta from mother to fetus, and some limited research indicates that it can cause birth defects. Germany's risk assessment agency warns pregnant women about the consumption of quinine-containing beverages. The labeling “contains quinine” is stated on every tonic or bitter lemon beverage. Although comprehensive research is still not available, it’s safer to completely avoid quinine-containing beverages during pregnancy.

Chapter 7: Other Freaky Data

Genetic defects, including Down syndrome, are definitely very scary. Every mom wishes for a healthy baby. And let's be honest, facing a future of dealing with a disabled child is nothing any parent desires. And Down syndrome in particular is the most common chromosome abnormality occurring in about 1 per 1000 babies born each year.

Since the occurrence of genetic abnormalities rises with the increasing age of parents, in many countries moms older than 30 are required to undertake genetic testing by their health insurance, including a procedure called *amniocentesis*. Amniocentesis involves inserting a needle through the uterus wall into the amniotic sac to acquire a sample of amniotic fluid for further testing. When I was pregnant with my first baby, I was already 36. It was highly recommended by my doctor to take the amniocentesis test, which I refused to do due to a potential risk of embryo damage. Now I'm 40, so I'm expecting my doctor will pressure me even more to undertake this procedure if I do become pregnant again. While I still have a choice [living in the

United States], my Czech gynecologist informed me that this procedure is mandatory for pregnant women over 35 in many European countries.

While I was looking up what's new in medical research, I came across a piece of news that made me smile: *New Blood Test Reliably Detects Down Syndrome and Other Genetic Abnormalities*. According to this new finding[8], routine screening using a non-invasive test that analyzes fetal DNA in a pregnant woman's blood can accurately detect Down syndrome and other genetic fetal abnormalities in the first trimester. This news could mean that by the time I'm in need of such screening, I might be able to avoid amniocentesis and still get accurate results on genetic abnormalities.

As I'm writing this, a very close friend just informs me that in her 11th week of pregnancy, they found a mutation of a Cystic fibrosis (CF) gene in her blood. That information totally freaks me out since we are about the same age and of similar genes. She explained that to determine the actual risk of the baby being affected by this genetic disorder, they also need to test the father. If the father tests positive for the same

---

[8] New blood test for Down syndrome and other genetic abnormalities

mutation, there is a high likelihood that the baby would be born with CF. The American College of Obstetricians and Gynecologists (ACOG) recommends testing for couples who have a personal or close family history of CF, and they recommend that carrier testing be offered to all Caucasian couples and be made available to couples of other ethnic backgrounds.

Great—what else is there to worry about before we even start?

Chapter 8: First Try

I'm freaking out a bit. My first menstrual period after the pill came only 24 days after the previous, so my first reaction is: "the pill messed me up!" After I talk to my gynecologist in Europe and my local one in the States, to my huge surprise, they deliver completely conflicting information. So to set the record straight, I do my own research from a few reputable sources and find something I really like.

"The good news about the Pill and pregnancy is that oral contraceptives can actually give you a boost in preserving your fertility by lowering your chances of getting uterine and ovarian cancer. It can also suppress the symptoms of endometriosis, in which the uterine lining grows outside the uterus, causing fertility problems. But can the Pill actually help you get pregnant after you stop using it? Not exactly. Even though some women who had erratic cycles swear that a few years on the Pill helped regulate them, doctors caution that the cycle regulation is artificial, and once women are off the Pill their fertility returns to whatever level it would have

been. Some women's cycles regulate themselves over time anyway, regardless of whether or not they take the Pill. Once you do decide to go off the Pill, finish up your monthly batch, and then prepare yourself to potentially becoming pregnant. Many doctors advise using a barrier method until you have had one or two periods, but that is only to help you keep track of your cycle so you can predict your due date. Even if you go off the Pill and get pregnant before you've had a period, a sonogram can help pinpoint how far along you are in your pregnancy."
From Parenting Magazine[9]

[9] How Birth Control Could Affect Your Fertility

Chapter 9: Considering in Vitro Fertilization?

As we say in Czech,
"You can't win a battle before fighting it first."

Several of my friends, including a cousin of mine, have undertaken the in vitro fertilization (IVF) procedure, but I have always felt a bit undecided about it. Not that there is anything wrong with getting some help if things don't work out naturally, especially at our age, but I'm still not 100% sure I would go through with it myself. I do have one child already, and all the cases I personally know of were trying for their first child after several unsuccessful attempts to conceive naturally. However, none of them was successful with the first IVF cycle, which made the following ones much more stressful and therefore riskier for success. And all these ladies were in their 30s, not their 40s like myself. Not to mention the cost: the American Society of Reproductive Medicine lists the average price of one IVF cycle at around $12,000. Now, if you are doing several cycles, it's a rather expensive procedure and almost a luxury for most women. Another aspect that should be mentioned is the physical, psychological and emotional impact this procedure may have on women due to sudden hormonal and other physiological changes to the body, adding extra stress on the couple as well.

But even with IVF, age still affects our chances of getting pregnant. Actually, according to the Society for Assisted Reproductive Technology (SART), woman's age is the most important factor influencing the success of IVF if she uses her own eggs. The success rate for women who are 32 and younger is around 40%, while for women who are 40 it's less than 20% and sharply declining after 40.

Considering the 5% chance of getting pregnant in any single ovulation cycle at this age, I think I'll give it a year before considering IVF. Be aware that it's often best to perform two IVF cycles (consecutive cycles usually run at half price)—unless one considers having the procedure done abroad in countries such as Mexico or the Czech Republic, where the treatment runs at about a quarter of the U.S. cost.

In either case, I would recommend doing your own research and verifying references before you make your choice. For younger women, there might be more choices coming soon as research continues and cheaper alternatives such as the "no-frills" IVF, which was introduced in the U.K. in 2014 and costs about 1,000 British pounds (cca $1,600), might be available.

Chapter 10: Parties and No Alcohol

As we say in Czech,

"A glass of wine won't kill you, and you won't be able to drink a whole barrel anyways."

"One drank and died; the other hadn't and died too."

My husband and I are pretty social people, and savoring alcohol is quite common in our circle of friends. Therefore, it's hard to keep saying you are on a "detox diet" even months after the holidays. Since I don't want to go around informing everybody that I'm trying to get pregnant, I have a small glass of wine every now and then, but keep it very low. We'll see how long I can get away with it. Of course, once I'm pregnant, I have no problem sharing my true reason, but not until then.

And what's the real deal with alcohol during pregnancy? Despite the fact that current medical evidence supporting strict abstinence from alcohol during pregnancy is not even very strong, most doctors will recommend it anyway, probably to play it safe.

However, several recent studies may raise a lot of discussion and controversy in this area. For example, a 2013 study by University College London researchers published in the *International Journal of Obstetrics and Gynaecology*[10] found that pregnant women who drink alcohol in moderation during the first trimester of pregnancy and possibly beyond are not putting their babies at risk for premature birth or low birth weight, or themselves at risk for high blood pressure complications during pregnancy.

Several other studies suggest that pregnant women who have an occasional drink won't harm themselves or their baby. For example, a 2012 research study from Denmark[11] found that low to moderate alcohol consumption during pregnancy did not affect executive functioning (activities such as planning, organizing, strategizing, remembering details, and managing time) among 5-year-olds.

---

[10] Light drinking during pregnancy is not linked to adverse behavioral or cognitive outcomes in childhood

[11] Danish studies suggest low and moderate drinking in early pregnancy has no adverse effects on children aged five

Another recent study from the University of Copenhagen[12] in Denmark found that children whose mothers drank moderately during pregnancy (about two drinks a week) experienced better mental health than children whose mothers completely abstained from drinking.

Since research is not yet clear how much alcohol it takes to cause any health problems, most experts still advice that women should avoid alcohol if they are pregnant or might become pregnant. However, women who were pregnant for a while before they discovered their pregnancy and consumed alcohol don't have to worry—their alcohol consumption likely didn't harm their unborn children.

Although many respected medical societies like the American College of Obstetricians and Gynecologists and the United Kingdom's Royal College of Obstetricians and Gynecologists urge women to abstain from any alcohol during pregnancy, some respected health agencies, such as the United Kingdom's Department of Health indicate that having one alcoholic beverage a couple times per week during pregnancy is okay.

---

[12] Prenatal exposure to alcohol, and gender differences on child mental health at age seven years

Chapter 11: Ovulation Kit

I never really worried about things like ovulation, let alone something like an ovulation reader. My first pregnancy came as a surprise, and I always thought we'd do it again. But since we decided to try for a girl now, ovulation time does matter, according to some. After I looked up ovulation calculators on Babycenter.com and ovulation-calendar.net, I feel pretty confident I have it down to a day, although their results are not exactly the same. Then a friend shows up with an ovulation kit, and my first reaction is, "What am I suppose to do with that?"

She looks at me as if I didn't know how to read and shrugs, "Dude, you pee on it and it will tell you whether you ovulate that day or not. And since you already have your fertility calendar, just do the test like 3 days in a row, and avoid sex on the ovulation day if you still want a girl."

All right, that sounds pretty easy. She had the kit unused from her last (and "final") pregnancy and thought it might come handy for me before it expires.

So here goes nothing. After I followed the instructions and my friend's advice exactly, the result was always negative. Well, maybe I just skipped ovulation that month, if that's even possible. Now we can have fun without stressing about performing "on call" and continue trying next month.

Chapter 12: Signs of Pregnancy?

Although ovulation didn't come last month, according to my smart ovulation reader, I still expect menstruation to come in plus-minus 28 days. Instead, on day 22, I have light bleeding. What the hell? Only two months after I gave up my pill, my period keeps coming in shorter and shorter intervals. I do some research on the subject and actually find that it's very common to get intervals longer than 30 days or even skipped several months, but nobody mentions such short periods. This time my bleeding only lasts a day, so I wait to see what would happen next.

Twenty-eight days later, and still nothing. Instead my breasts hurt and feel somewhat swollen, I have shortness of breath, and I feel really tired. Must be the spring! I decide to do a home pregnancy test anyways, just to be sure. I dig one out from my medicine cabinet, but it's already 2 years expired. Hmm, shall I still use it? How bad could it be! The worst-case scenario it simply won't work. Here we go. I receive a solid line in each window. Problem is, I don't have the instruction box anymore, so how do I read the results?

Back to the computer. While my super-active 3-year old is watching the Curious George cartoon, I'm searching through pictures of all existing home test devices, looking for the one that looks like mine. Bingo! And the news is that it reads "positive." Really? And now what!

Chapter 13: How to Deal with the News

Now that there is a first indication of good news, the real worry begins. Yes, you are 40 after all, so anything can go wrong at any given moment for any possible reason. If you share your news with your friends right away, you might receive a shopping list of NO-NOs and constant reminders of what to eat, what to do, and how to take it easy all the time. I'm going to give myself a break from all of that and simply won't tell anybody until things are confirmed and somewhat more "secured."

The next step is to find myself a good doctor since I'm new in town and I haven't had a chance to find one yet. My current general doctor is amazing. She gives me thumbs up, assuring me that urine pregnancy tests are pretty accurate, and if anything, they would show negative results for a positive condition but never the other way around. She inscribes a long referral for all sorts of blood tests so we can verify my new condition as well as my state of health. That will give me enough information while I'm searching for the right doctor, and my generalist is willing to consult me on all my results until I land one. I feel sort of relieved, not only she's a woman and a mom herself, she's about my age and super cool. She reminds me of my Czech gynecologist who I can discuss anything with and never get a stare or a disapproving look, as I experienced with many previous doctors.

Chapter 14: So Now That You Are Pregnant at 40, What's Next?

I can't quite say whether I'm happy or concerned about this new finding. Obviously, I don't accept the positive result until it's verified by a more accurate blood test, but it does make me think about it a lot.

The next day, I head out for my blood and urine tests with an empty stomach. I absolutely hate fasting since I get dizzy very easily if I don't eat within 30 minutes after getting up (courtesy of my anemia and low blood pressure). In the lab they take all the blood and urine they need, so I can finally have my breakfast and feel "normal." Since I was sick a lot as a child and spent some time in hospitals (thanks to contracting Scarlet fever at the age of 4 and then again 14 months later, which left me with a lot of ongoing health issues), blood drawing doesn't make my stomach turn and I can watch it with ease.

Three days later, which happens to be Friday, all my results with the exception of one are ready. For whatever reason (probably lack of brain oxygenation), it doesn't even cross my mind to ask if I could collect them now and get the missing one later, and I simply agree to wait till Monday. On Monday, they tell me it hasn't arrived yet and maybe I can check in another 2 to 3 days. Once again, it doesn't cross my mind to ask if I could collect the majority of them now and the missing one later. Maybe somehow subconsciously I didn't want to know the results—who knows. But the lab assistant doesn't suggest it either, which makes me think that nobody involved is using their brains as they should, even at work.

I finally stop by the lab on Wednesday and sure enough—the missing result is still not there. This time I'm taking all the others and will continue waiting for the last one, which is an estrogen test, rather important one too. The results show positive pregnancy and hormone levels indicate gestational progress of about 5–6 weeks. Wow. All my other life essentials are almost book-perfect, except for an increased hyperthyroid and therefore a shortage of CO2 in my blood. Well, it could have definitely been much worse.

Chapter 15: Bleeding

My close friend from New York is visiting me for a few days, and I'm taking some time off to enjoy her company and to catch up, especially since we now have some new things to talk about. We enjoy a day at the beach with some virgin pina coladas and lots of laughter. Later that day, I notice a dark blood stain on my bathing suit. That's definitely strange, but maybe that's just a one-time event. I don't pay much attention to it until it happens again the next day. I call my "pregnancy advisor" dula-friend. She assures me that if it's dark blood, it's not a real-time bleeding, and therefore it's nothing to worry about. It might be implantation bleeding, or a ruptured small blood vessel, but definitely nothing to lose your sleep over. She recommends getting another HCG hormone[13] analysis done just to make sure the levels are still rising, which translates to a "live fetus." Coincidently, the same day, I get a call from the lab, that the analyzing lab ran out of my blood and needs another tube to finish the last test.

---

[13] HCG or human chorionic gonadotropin, the pregnancy hormone

Once again I visit the lab, and I ask them if they could run another HCG test as well. I can provide them with another doctor referral before the results come in. They know me by now and trust my word. Good work, everybody!

It's Friday afternoon and according to the latest published research from Harvard Medical School, one glass of wine a week is absolutely acceptable during pregnancy, and reportedly beneficial for the baby's mental health, so I will definitely savor this one with my visitors and enjoy the weekend. The bleeding doesn't seem to completely go away during the weekend; even when it stops, it comes back the next day or later at night. Everybody is calming me down, saying that it's nothing serious unless it's an oxygenated bright red blood. It definitely stays on my mind, and this time I can't wait to get my results on Monday. New results indicate that everything is fine, HCG levels rising, so I can relax until I see my doctor for a full examination.

Chapter 16: Getting a Doctor

One would think that in the 21st century, getting a doctor in a civilized world should not be a problem. But getting a good doctor is often a big challenge, and might require some trials before you find the right match. What never occurred to me was that getting a doctor once pregnant might be harder or even impossible—probably comparable to getting health insurance in the U.S. once you are seriously sick or pregnant for that matter.

After two scheduled appointments and numerous phone calls, I realize there are only two gynecologists in my area that actually "do pregnancies"; and as anybody can imagine, they must be pretty busy. The first office never picks up the phone, and the other office invites me to stop by to fill out a "screening form," based on which the doctor would either give me an appointment or not. Another office gives me an appointment based on the fact that I'm pregnant; however, after I show up and wait for an hour to see the doctor, the nurse tells me that the doctor doesn't do pregnancies anymore. What? The one doctor I really want to see, who also comes highly recommended, doesn't do twins or high-risk pregnancies. Am I considered a high-risk pregnancy since I'm 40 now? That really gets me going.

That night, I email my gynecologist in Europe who I've been seeing since college and who I always visit when I am "back home." I reveal my whole situation to her and concern over the bleeding that has been going on for over a week now. Her immediate response —I mean, she responds only 3 hours after I email her at 1am her time—is quite alarming. She instructs me to get a sonogram immediately to verify what's going on with the pregnancy since repeated bleeding during the first trimester can mean many different things; some of them serious. Now I'm really freaking out.

The next day, I try to call my general doctor to get a referral for a sonogram, but nobody is answering the phone all morning. I'm aware that she also works at the emergency room, and it happened before that she simply didn't show up for her regular hours because she was stuck in a surgery or with an urgent case.

"She's not in, really?" I ask the receptionist to double confirm. So I call my sonogram lab and ask if they would do a sonogram for me if I supplied a referral later. The radiologist recommends I go to an emergency room instead and have a doctor evaluate my condition, including all necessary tests and a sonogram. At this point, I'm not waiting any longer and head for the nearest hospital, which has a reputation of being crowded 24/7. "Just take a deep breath," I remind myself.

To my huge surprise (and based on my previous experience in that emergency hospital), I get attended to by a doctor within an hour after my arrival, in the next 30 minutes they take my blood and urine samples to run the necessary tests, and in the following hour I have a sonogram done. Wow, I hardly even had time to read a book! When all results come back, about 3 hours after I arrived, the doctor explains that everything looks absolutely normal, the baby is alive and well, and I have nothing to worry about. But he does order bed rest. Bed rest? What am I sick or what? "How long?" I ask.

"Until you see your doctor who can instruct you further," he replies. Well, it's all good news, I guess, but I don't even have a doctor, so my bed rest is infinite for now.

As I'm getting ready to check out, a phone

rings, and a nurse from the new doctor (the one I actually hoped for) calls to give me an appointment. Great! But it's not for another 2 weeks. Oh well, at least I know I won't be "resting" forever, not that I can even visualize what a "bed rest" really translates to.

Chapter 17: Before My First Doctor Visit

The following two weeks are a bit of a self-induced hell. Not only does the bleeding keep appearing and disappearing at random times, but my sort of "morning sickness" goes on all day, and I usually don't feel better until it's bedtime when I'm drop-dead exhausted to make up for the lost time. So my days sort of drag along, between light activities, resting, and feeling like crap. Being a total foodie, to my huge surprise, I have no appetite at all. And although I eat quite often, the enjoyment is not quite there. Some things that I normally really indulge in, such as dark chocolate, cheese, arugula, or cilantro, are almost making me gag. That makes me even more miserable since there isn't much left for me to enjoy.

Chapter 18: First Doctor's Visit

I did indeed survive those long 2 weeks of anticipation, and the bleeding has disappeared completely. As a good and well-mannered girl, I arrive to my 11 am appointment 5 minutes early, just to make sure I'm on time. The front door is locked with a big sign that says "CLOSED." What? A lovely middle-aged lady explains that they open at 11 am, so not to stress. Do I look stressed? I guess so. I sit down on a bench outside the entrance and try to look relaxed.

At 11 am, a nurse arrives and lets us (me and the middle-aged lady) inside the waiting room. She doesn't say a word and starts organizing her desk behind the teller window. The lovely middle-aged lady walks in and stops at a "privacy line" and patiently waits to be asked to approach the window. That doesn't happen for another 5 minutes while I just sit there wondering what's next. Once other people start arriving, I get up too and stand right behind her, waiting to see what happens. The nurse finally asks the lovely middle-aged lady to step up to the window and to my surprise they are done in a minute. Now it's my turn. Alright, I have to sign papers, lots of papers, most of them I'm not even reading, as it gives me a headache and it needs to be done regardless. Then I'm asked to take a seat and wait to be called. While I was signing all these papers, the room has filled up with another 10, mostly young women, some with children, some with partners. So I take out my current book and focus on the story to take my mind off the subject. After some time I'm asked in by another nurse to be weighed and have my blood pressure taken. "The doctor is not here yet, but you are the first patient he'll be seeing today," the nurse tells me after she collects all my personal data.

"When are you expecting him?" I ask, looking at my watch, which shows 12.

She shrugs her shoulders: "You know he also works at the hospital so if there's an emergency, he has to attend it. But he usually comes to his office right after." Wow, I think to myself. He's got a waiting room full of anxious women who are expected just to sit there and wait until he shows up. "But you can pay now for your first visit and the lab tests so you don't have to do that later," she says with a smile. Of course I will. That's why I'm here, right? Just pay and wait.

"Could I step outside to get some lunch and

come back in half an hour? I didn't expect to be waiting here that long and I'm quite hungry already."

The nurse responds affirmatively.

I return happy with a full stomach; in the meantime, the waiting room has exploded with female patients and their male companions. The nurse has been looking for me already and I'm asked to come right in and into the doctor's office. This must have been the first time I'm at a doctor's office that looks like a lawyer's office. Maybe I'm stereotyping, but I always associated dark mahogany furniture with granite tabletops and dark leather armchairs with people of power: lawyers, politicians or bankers, but not doctors. I guess he's doing very well then. Where is the exam table? Are we supposed to sign more papers or discuss some theory? He sits me down opposite from him and starts interviewing me—the usual medical stuff. He then proceeds to ask about my religion. Really!? And then he asks about the number of partners I have been with. That certainly throws me off. I'm 40 years old and had all sorts of doctors in my adult life, but this is the very first time somebody has inquired and asked me about an exact number. Shouldn't the question be more like: "Are you practicing safe sex? If not, have you had any STDs and which?" Hmm, shall I say the truth or not?

The doctor realizes I'm hesitating, so he adds: "Less than five or more?"

"More than five," I answer, relieved.

Then we move to the exam room with the usual stirrup table and a sonogram machine next to it. The doctor is very professional and gently performs an intra-vaginal sonogram exam. I eagerly watch the monitor for a familiar image. "Here it is," he smiles. "Here is your uterus and here is our little buddy. This here is the heart, which sounds good. Let's do some measurements. Yes, the measurements correspond with just about 9 weeks. Everything looks very good now, but we are still in the risky period, so for the next few weeks I would recommend you take it really easy—no sex, no excessive exercise, and we'll check again in about 3 weeks."

I feel content and ask what he thinks about the light bleeding I experienced earlier. He just shrugs his shoulders, says that it could have been anything, but the baby is fine and unless the bleeding returns or I experience any other complications, everything should be fine. Then he gives me referral for lab work to check my antibodies for rubella and HIV, STDs, and a urine analysis—anything that could affect the healthy course of my pregnancy. He also takes a pap smear to test for HPV and cervical cancer.

"And we are all done. Take it easy and see you in 3 weeks," as he shakes my hand.

Chapter 19: From 9 to 12 Weeks

Alright, I know I should take it easy, and I'm really trying hard. But I'm not the type who can just sit around reading books all day. I do have a very active and busy life, so "taking it easy" in my dictionary means that I won't carry any bricks around, I might replace running with fast walking, and I will try not to stress too much. But that's about as much as I'm willing to compromise. Plus, I do have 3 businesses, a 3-year old, a house, big garden, and lots of projects that are constantly developing. At the same time, I realize that the first 12 weeks are the most risky and vulnerable to miscarriage, especially at my age. So I guess I should seek some kind of a happy medium.

Chapter 20: Surfing

Although surfing is not my obsession, I do enjoy it. With my busy schedule and a family, I don't get to surf very much, but once a week with my girlfriends is a nice treat. During the winter, the waves tend to be bigger, so I normally pick and choose, and especially now—given my risky period—I'm very, very careful and only go out when it's quite small and easy. Truth be told, I haven't surfed much during this pregnancy so far, probably a handful of times during the past 12 weeks or so, and it has always been very mellow.

At this age, I prefer to be safe than sorry. Other girls in my community don't seem to share the same opinion. I can understand that if you are an experienced or professional surfer, you are more in control than, say, myself, but I have a problem seeing a future mom with a huge belly paddling into 6-foot waves. Some of them even surfed until their 6th month of pregnancy, including Hawaiian pro-surfer Bethany Hamilton, who on top of being pregnant only has one arm after a shark attacked her few years back. That I consider very foolish and irresponsible. But it's solely my personal opinion. I'm happy none of them (that I know of) had any accidents or problems with their pregnancies as a result of surfing.

Being a competitive athlete who has always indulged in dangerous sports, I would personally not recommend practicing anything risky, especially during the later stages of pregnancy.

Chapter 21: Second Doctor's Visit

I have been a good girl for the past three weeks, and I'm really looking for some good news today that will give me peace of mind. I have also not told anyone about my pregnancy (other than my husband), and we are both now ready to tell our parents and close friends. My appointment is not until after lunch, and although my husband orders me to take it easy and not do anything, I can't just sit around being useless. I feel well enough, and today is Thursday, which in my household translates to a cleaning day. I spend the entire morning cleaning the house, and then I have a nice and nutritious lunch and decide to call the office to confirm my appointment. The nurse informs me that due to a doctor's emergency and hospital duties, my appointment has to be postponed until 3 pm. Somehow, I expected that. Although I have time to do some more work, I put my feet up and read a book instead. I'm not much of a reader, but this book called *The Storyteller* by Jodi Picoult really got my attention, and I don't feel an ounce of guilt reading now while I should be doing more work.

At 3 pm on the dot, I check in with the receptionist and go right in. After a routine weight and blood pressure check performed by the nurse, I'm asked right into the exam room and up the stirrup table. I can't wait to see the baby grown and more developed now at 12 weeks. The doctor greets me and says a joke to make me smile while turning his ultrasound scanner on. "How have you been feeling? Did the bleeding stop? Anything unusual?"

"Everything is fine," I reply. "The bleeding hasn't come back since my last visit. I have just been feeling very tired, but have followed your orders otherwise."

He gives me a smile: "Excellent. So let's check the baby's heart beat and look how he's doing."

I smile back and turn my head toward the monitor. He runs the scanner over my belly, points to a small stretch mark, and turns his head toward the monitor. Then he brings the sound up and focuses on the sounds that are coming out. But there's nothing that would resemble a heartbeat. I try to read his face, as he's not saying a word while checking again. Then he touches my underbelly gently and asks me to empty my bladder in the bathroom so we can do a vaginal sonogram to take a closer look. He doesn't say or explain anything else just asks me to use the toilet and says we'll continue after.

I run to the bathroom, feeling a cold sweat come over me. I don't quite know what to think, but I don't have a good feeling. During the few minutes I spend in the bathroom, my thoughts are all over the place: "Have I done something wrong in the last three weeks? Is the sonogram possibly not working properly? Am I ready to hear what the doctor has to say?" Although I want to extend the time thinking about all these things, I return briskly back to the exam room, and sit on the table waiting. Instinctively, I touch my belly, and although I'm not religious at all, I find myself asking for good news. At the same time, I'm running another scenario in my head, and that is, if the news is not good, will I be able to become pregnant again at this age? How long will it take me? The time is running out for me. Then I tell myself to take a deep breath and accept whatever the news is as a new reality.

The doctor and nurse both re-enter, and now I'm really anxiously waiting to see the monitor. As he inserts the scanner and starts moving it in search of my uterus, I feel my heart racing. All three of us are now staring at the monitor as the image of my uterus with the baby appears. Mixed feelings flood my brain. We can clearly see there is a baby there, but there doesn't seem to be any motion or heartbeat detectable. The doctor measures the fetus and comments that it's quite small. I don't quite remember now if I have actually asked him a question or if we communicated non-verbally, but we both knew what that meant. He asks me to get dressed and meet him in his office. I'm trying to breathe and control my emotions. When we sit down, he tells me that he needs to have another sonogram done to verify his findings today since there's always a possibility of an equipment malfunction. However, the sonogram image he has printed corresponds to a fetus size of 9 weeks. He explains that when the fetus stops developing or dies, often due to genetic abnormalities, it starts shrinking in size, while the mother's body still functions like if it's carrying a live baby. I ask him what usually happens after the fetus dies since it seems it might have happened already a few weeks ago.

"Your body might start recognizing the baby has died and will start the process of removal on its own. This can happen tomorrow or it may take weeks. You can either let it go naturally or we could schedule a procedure for ITS[14] removal. But let's discuss that once

---

[14] It's interesting how we sometimes refer to human fetuses. We can find references in professional literature

we have confirmation that the pregnancy has really been aborted."

Then he gives me a referral for another sonogram and asks me to return as soon as I have my results to discuss what we will do next. "Just in case you start bleeding over the next few days, I want you go to the ER right away."

I nod in agreement and storm out of the office and onto the street so nobody can see what my face is expressing. Once I'm sitting in my car, I start crying uncontrollably.

---

calling the fetus IT, but we can also find references calling the fetus a little HE or SHE, especially in doctors' offices. Clearly, that's a more emotional approach that future parents feel comfortable with. So what happens when the fetus dies? Is it okay to change the reference from HE/SHE to IT? How does that make the future mom feel, when in the blink of an eye, it's not her little he, she, or a baby inside her body, but just a thing, some object, that's there when it shouldn't be there anymore?

Chapter 22: Reality Check

As we say in Czech,

"The more you cry, the less you pee."

Even with all the known risk factors pregnancy after 40 carries, none of us who are planning on having a baby at this age want to believe it will happen to us. Conceiving might seem to be the biggest challenge here, but losing a baby once we have conceived naturally and without any problems is hard to accept. Yet, the data speak quite clearly, and torturing ourselves by obsessing over all the possible *if's* is definitely not the way to go.

The next day, I visit another sonogram place, where they confirm what my doctor had found the day before. The examining doctor suggests I take it super easy over the weekend (since it's Friday) to avoid possible rupture of the embolic sac, which could lead to severe hemorrhaging. I'm happy my husband is with me there, and although I do cry again, I think this visit helps me with closure, instead of waiting until Monday to verify this new reality. My husband and I go to pick our 3-year old up from his daycare together, which hardly happens since our schedules are so different. Our toddler is in a great mood and can't wait to take us both to play in the park. So we go. When we get home, I suggest to my husband that we open a bottle of wine to take my mind off the subject and relax a bit. Good wine always helps.

Chapter 23: Weekend Emergency

Like a good girl, I follow the doctor's and my husband's instructions and do absolutely nothing (except for eating and reading an "inspiring" holocaust book). Then on Saturday afternoon, when everybody is napping, I start bleeding. At first, I stay totally calm and just observe what's going to happen during the next hour or so. The bleeding doesn't stop, and although it isn't too strong, we decide we better go to the hospital now, rather than in the middle of the night. Coincidentally, that evening we had planned for our son's first sleepover party at my friend's house, so we drop him off a bit earlier and head out for the ER.

Although the waiting room isn't crowded and I'm admitted rather fast, I end up waiting on a stretcher in a hallway for almost 2 hours before the doctor-in-charge attends me. After observing him walking around all this time, I'm almost ready to bail; he seems a bit out there. His unusually thin figure as well as his mannerism reminds me of *don Quixote de la Mancha.* His sunken cheekbones and empty eyes are almost frightening. He reeks of cigarettes and maybe he has been drinking (a bit) too, suggesting the stressful life of an ER doctor. After he listens to my story with his ear about 12 inches from my mouth, he orders lab work, another sonogram, and tells me he will contact my gynecologist to determine the next step. However, by the time all the results come in, it's already 11 pm. I realize nothing is going to happen that day unless I'm seriously hemorrhaging. But at least I want to get an appointment for the fetus removal procedure now, instead of more waiting at my gynecologist's office on Monday afternoon.

As expected, my gynecologist offers two scenarios (via cell phone from his bedroom). To be honest, I'm a bit surprised that one of the options is simply to wait until my body takes care of the business and flushes the dead fetus out on its own. The second option is an emergency D&C procedure (dilation and curettage) on Monday morning, during which the doctor would remove the dead fetus surgically under general anesthesia. Since I had done my research already, my answer is quick and simple: D&C. I'm released with instructions not to eat or drink anything after midnight on Sunday and show up back at the ER on Monday at 6 am.

The next morning (Sunday), I pick our son up from his sleepover party, and the 3 of us spend the day doing nothing. Actually, in our family language that translates to: my husband goes to surf, I make banana pancakes for breakfast, and when my husband returns, we spend the rest of the morning at our neighbor's pool playing and swimming. Although it's been a very relaxing day, all I want is to have the removal procedure over with and move on. There is still one little detail, which has to be resolved: my procedure is scheduled for early Monday morning, and since it's going to be performed under general or full anesthesia, I won't be able to drive myself home after. So my husband has to go with me, which means that somebody has to be with our son when we leave at 5:30 am. As much as I don't want to get anybody else involved, we have to call my husband's mom and explain the situation. Of course, she has no idea I was pregnant; we were planning to tell her on Mother's day at 14 weeks. She's very supportive and has no problem sleeping over on Sunday and taking care of our son in the morning, which includes dropping him off at his daycare.

Chapter 24: D&C

Right around 6 am, we arrive at the hospital and inquire about my admission at the emergency room, just like we were told on Saturday night. The emergency room is entirely empty and the desk clerk is still half asleep after her night shift, but she explains that for scheduled surgeries we have to check in at the main admission desk. So we sign my name on the list and wait. About 30 minutes later, a nurse calls my name and asks for my admission referrals. When I explain my full story and say we were told my admission documents would be ready here from Saturday night, she rolls her eyes and says we need to go back to the emergency check-in, as there isn't anything with my name on file there. So we do as we are told. We proceed with the usual emergency admission paperwork and are asked to wait. It's little after 7 am and the waiting room starts to fill up. While the sun is shining outside, it's a freeze box inside the ER. Despite my preparedness—I brought a warm jacket with a hood, wool socks, and warm blanket—I'm still shivering from the cold. This time the wait is quite long, although it appeared I was the very first patient there.

Close to 8 am, I'm getting quite anxious; I'm really cold, hungry, and thirsty, but I'm not allowed to ingest anything because of the anesthesia. I could have slept another 2 hours if I knew I would be waiting this long. My husband just smiles at my naivety: "Didn't you expect this based on our previous experiences?" I guess I was naïve, thinking I would be back home for lunch.

Shortly after, I'm called in and placed in one of their cubicles. The head nurse explains they will prepare me for the surgery with an IV now and as soon as the doctor arrives, I will be wheeled in. "Sounds good to me," I think to myself and look at my husband smiling. Then two very young girls—probably nurses in training—arrive and the head nurse starts to explain how to tap an artery and how to insert the flexible needle. The young girl struggles to insert the needle in my artery and after a few unsuccessful tries, she asks the head nurse to help her. That did it for me. I start weeping—not from the pain, but from exhaustion and self-pity, I guess. Unfortunately, the adventure is far from being over.

Soon after, I'm wheeled over to the pre-operation room, where I'm asked to undress completely and put on a disposable gown for the surgery and continue waiting. And this room is a real freezer. Unless I'm so tired by now that I'm shivering even under the warm blanket. One hour into my waiting, I overhear somebody in the background mentioning that my doctor has arrived and is getting ready for his first surgery. When I ask the supervising nurse if that means I will go into surgery soon, she replies the doctor hasn't arrived yet and he has one other patient before me. It's about 11 am. My husband receives a pager and instructions from the head nurse, and I send him home so he can focus on his work instead of waiting. Then I take out my holocaust book and continue reading, realizing I might finish the entire book before it's my turn. About 10 people come through the pre-operation room and are taken to surgery before another doctor approaches and informs me that I will soon go to surgery under a full anesthesia. He has me sign bunch of papers I don't even bother reading. I only found out later in the operation room that he is my anesthesiologist; he must have forgotten to mention such an important detail. Soon after, another nurse dressed in winter jacket comes over and wheels me into a hallway, just outside several surgery rooms. At this point, I don't even bother asking when I'm going in and continue with my book.

At about noon, a doctor with a surgical mask approaches and calls me by my name. I don't recognize him at first, but then I realize it's my gynecologist. He asks how I'm feeling, how strong is the bleeding now, and informs me that I'm his next patient. But he first needs to explain the risks of D&C and have me sign more papers. I can't help myself and remind him that both he and the sonogram doctor warned me about possible serious hemorrhaging and recommended that I go to the ER immediately if bleeding occurs. Therefore, I did and I was sent home and requested to be here today at 6 am. He agrees that it‘s the right and safe thing to do, and even if I had decided to wait for the body to remove the dead fetus on its own, we might have needed the procedure later on anyways to make sure everything was cleared properly. However, he has to warn me about the possible risks this procedure carries, such as that under extreme circumstances, they would have to remove my uterus completely. My eyes must have grown so large at that sentence that he immediately backs off and assures me that's not going to happen, but I still have to sign the paper anyways. At this point, I'm so weak and tired and just want it to be over no matter what.

So when they finally bring me to the operation room, about 6.5 hours later, I really try to relax. The assisting nurses are teasing me how unusually tall and skinny I am that they have to adjust the operating table just for me, and they entertain themselves by guessing my accent and origin. My gynecologist is meanwhile receiving several phone calls from his office. He has patients scheduled and waiting there already, but he won't be able to be there for at least another hour. Before I go to sleep, I turn to him and ask jokingly not to rush this surgery since I'm still planning on using my uterus in the near future. That's the last thing I remember.

I wake up some time later in the pre-surgery room with my husband by my side.

Chapter 25: It's Party Time

Now that I'm not pregnant anymore, maybe I should enjoy life again a bit more (not that I don't enjoy it already, but mamas out there know what I mean). Mother's Day is coming in a few days and I'm feeling good. And not that I want to go on a binge, but I will gladly enjoy more than one glass of good wine with my dinner now.

It's Sunday afternoon, a week after the procedure. Our little boy is spending time with his grandma, so my husband and I can take a little break from the recent craziness. We are chilling in our lovely tropical garden with some Pinot Noir and talking about our upcoming trip to Europe. It will be a nice distraction and a perfect time to heal, both physically and emotionally. My husband mentions he has never been to Italy, probably one of the few places he hasn't visited in Europe.

"Really? Then what about Northern Italy, we could fly to Milano from Prague and travel from there," I suggest.

Then all of a sudden I get really sentimental and tears start coming down my cheeks. I can't explain how or why, it's simply happening. I suppose my hormones are all over the place now.

He notices my unexpected transformation and touches my hand gently: "How are you feeling?"

I look back at him and smile through my tears. I've always had a problem hiding my emotions; my face is like a mirror of my mind, for better or for worse. As much as I'm trying, I can't just easily erase the whole episode from my head. "Did you ever wonder if it was a boy or a girl?" I ask.

He's looking at me in silence with his mouth half open, as if he was racing for the right words in his head. I smile at him clearing my tears. "I know I should just let it go."

"Of course I did," he responds. But neither one of us did anything wrong, and it happened for a reason. You know that!"

"I know", I reply. "Well, let's hope we'll do a better job next time, mister," I wink at him, smiling as more tears start coming down.

Chapter 26: Tooth Infection

As we say in Czech, "If you have a flu and treat it, it will take you about a week to recover. If you let be, it will take you about 7 days."

Everything seems to be healing fine, my bleeding stopped 5 days after the D&C procedure, and I feel good. It's time to go back to my regular routine of morning runs and get in shape. This morning, as I'm doing my oral hygiene routine, I notice that the gum area surrounding my root canal is a bit swollen. That's not too surprising since 3 days ago I woke up with an intense clench in my jaw, as if I was pushing on my lower teeth all night in stress or pain. I must have irritated that area so much that it got inflamed. Since I don't have any pain, a little icing and Ibuprofen should do the trick.

But the following day, I notice a little bump on top of the swollen area, as though an infection is building. I still don't feel any pain, so I decide to wait and see what happens.

The third day I accidentally poke into the bump with my toothbrush and white puss pours out. Ouch, that is clearly an infection. It's Friday evening and my dentist won't be reachable until tomorrow. I soak a Q-tip into tee tree oil (which disinfects the area and also works as antiseptic), squeeze the remainder of the puss out, and clean the entire area. Everything looks good, and I don't feel any pain at all.

The next day, I keep calling my dentist's office, but nobody is picking up. And although it's Saturday, I know the office is open until noon. I decide to go there in person, and to my surprise the office is really closed. Second ouch, as I realize they won't reopen until Tuesday afternoon. And now what!? I have 3 days to deal with a tooth infection, and the prospect that I might need to go to the ER again makes me really cringe. I'm trying to keep cool and think of grandma's old remedies. Plumb brandy, aka *Slivovitz*. So I prescribe myself another drainage of the infection by squeezing it out using a Q-tip dipped in tee tree oil and gargling and rinsing my mouth 3 times a day with the delicious plumb brandy I store for "unique occasions" to kill the bacteria in my mouth and limiting them from entering my stomach.

On Tuesday afternoon, my dentist looks at my swollen bump (which is half the size by now) and calls his assistant to show her the “enormous” abscess. “This is most likely coming from your root canal tooth, which might have a fracture. Let’s get an X-ray and take a look, okay?” Then he storms out to the neighboring room to attend another patient.

His assistant, who attended me few weeks earlier and knew about my pregnancy, looks at me all bewildered and says: “Why didn’t you tell him that you are pregnant and shouldn’t be exposed to X-rays?” “Because I’m not pregnant anymore,” I reply. She looks at me sadly and puts a heavy apron over my chest. “I’m really sorry to hear that!”

When the doctor returns and looks at the negative, he bites his lips: “It needs to go.”

I turn around, looking at him questionably. “Look over here,” he points to the X-ray picture. “There is a tiny fracture right here on the root, but since it’s a dead tooth, we can’t fix it, so it must be extracted.”

I start sweating like crazy. That’s definitely not the answer I expected.

"I'll open and clean it up now and give you antibiotics, but I would recommend that you take care of this right away. I mean, I can schedule you for Friday, by then the abscess should be gone." I stay silent, not knowing what to say. Then I come back to my senses and realize that I have a long trip ahead of me the following week. Should I wait to have the extraction or not? The idea of losing a baby and a tooth forever, and all in the scope of 10 days, is still a bit of a harsh reality for me.

Chapter 27: Tooth Extraction and Birthday Party

Right when I get emotionally prepared for the latest upcoming loss and schedule myself for Friday, it gets postponed for Saturday due to somebody's emergency. But Saturday is a birthday party for my boy's best friend, and there is no way we can miss it. Most moms would agree with me that you don't mess with kid's birthday parties, so pain or not, we have to attend. Since I'm scheduled for 10 am, I should be feeling fine by 3 pm. Although, something tells me this is not going to be on time anyways.

On Saturday, by the time I actually go in, it's about noon, and when I get out it's way past 1 pm. Great, my mouth is completely numb and bleeding, I'm a bit dizzy from all the drilling and pulling and I have only 2 hours to get over it. Just suck it up, girl!

By 3 pm, I still have gauze tucked in the new crater and I'm spitting blood every 10 minutes, but I feel okay. The anesthetic has faded away by now, and surprisingly, I have no pain at all.

At the party, despite the huge turnout, I seem to be the center of attention, mainly among the adults. Everybody is asking what happened to me and what a trooper I am to show up at a kid's birthday party in such condition. I'm trying to smile, but that actually hurts a bit and makes me bleed more. So I'm attempting to have some form of conversation while biting on my bloody gauze. Then my stomach kicks in: "I'm hungry!" Great. Of course, I haven't eaten anything since breakfast and I'm starving. There is no baby food around, I shouldn't be drinking alcohol yet, and I can't bite on anything. All I can do is mush some watermelon and bananas and keep pushing the tiny pieces through the corner of my mouth with unusual patience. Hopefully I can soon have some alcohol to make up for the frustrations and pain.

Chapter 28: High-Risk HPV Infection

If I were superstitious, I would say bad things usually come in 3's. First, I lose my baby, then a tooth, so what's coming next? I really hope this is it for a while. Two days after I arrive to visit my parents in my hometown, I go to see my local gynecologist, who has been my doctor since my early 20s. Since I didn't get a chance to see my current gynecologist after the procedure, I want her to check if everything is healing well and if I still have my uterus for that matter (kidding, I think). I love my local doctor. Not only is she a very worldly, modern woman, she has a good sense of humor and always responds promptly to my emergency email requests, even though she's not obligated to do so. I feel very comfortable talking to her about any sensitive matter.

On my visit, she first takes some tissue samples from my cervix to be analyzed for cytology and HPV, as she does on every single visit. Then she examines me with her colposcope and sonogram. Everything looks good and clean, except for some suspicious white spots on my cervix. I ask her about trying for another baby since opinions differ tremendously among different doctors. She acknowledges that new research leans toward shorter periods after a D&C than previously deemed healthy (6 months or more), but she still recommends waiting 3 menstrual cycles for the uterus to heal properly after the procedure.

"If you had a spontaneous removal of the deceased fetus, you could get pregnant without waiting, but since there might be some scar tissue, it's safer to heal properly so the next baby has the right environment to develop in," she explains. That makes perfect sense to me; still I'm not necessarily going to follow her advice.

A week later, I bump into her while shopping near my home. She's in her shorts with a huge dog on a leash, and I pass right by her without taking any notice of her. She calls my name, and when I turn around it takes me few seconds to recognize her. "Hi, I have good news about your cytology; it's absolutely normal. We still have to wait for the HPV analysis, so call me next week." I barely have a chance to respond and she's gone.

The telephone call that follows our meeting isn't as uplifting. She informs me that the lab analysis returned positive findings on several types of the HPV virus. Thankfully, the two strains that could lead to cervical cancer—type 16 and 18—are negative; however, given the viral persistence over the last decade, she wants me to see a specialist to get an opinion. That phone call totally puts me in a weird mood, understandably. I'm only staying in Europe for 3 more weeks, but I'm planning to have a little vacation away from home, so that gives me a very small window for the exam. And as I'm told, the recommended two hospitals that have real experts perform this ambulatory examination only twice a week. My consecutive calls for an appointment confirm that the earliest I could have this exam done is in 2 months. That means I have to deal with this back home in the U.S. This makes things a bit complicated. Not only do American and European experts use different analytical tools, they also often differ or even contradict each other with their opinions. Not to mention the cost; while in the EU it would cost me a small administrative fee of about two dollars, in the U.S. it will cost about $150 with good health insurance. But there is no other option; I need to get an expert to evaluate the results, perform a biopsy, and determine the best solution. There's another factor I need to mention, and that is the fact that I'll be trying to get pregnant again soon. Although there isn't currently any research that could scientifically confirm this fact, childbirth could help the body to cleanse and rid itself of the infection. That's exactly what happened to me after my first delivery—I had no virus indication for 3.5 years.

Chapter 29: Second Try at Making a Baby

As we say in Czech,

"Measure twice, cut only once."

Like a good girl, I follow the instructions of my Czech doctor and wait 3 menstrual cycles before trying to get pregnant again. Now, that we are in the "clear," it's time to get back to work. This time, I'm not worrying about conceiving a girl or a boy; there's absolutely no pressure and we'll see what happens. Still I have to admit, that "scheduled baby making" is a job like any other, and the reason to have sex is rarely pleasure—maybe because subconsciously (and perhaps even consciously) you think about the outcome rather than the process, so there is a certain level of stress involved. A friend, who is my age and has been trying to get pregnant for couple of years now, has compared "scheduled baby making" to playing the lottery or investing in the stock market. My supportive girlfriends keep telling me, "At least you'll have fun with it, and see what happens." Yeah right. The reality is quite different, especially at this age, when you know your time is really limited.

A few weeks go by, and it's time again for my next period. It's Saturday, and we have a beach party. I've stopped using tampons completely and now I'm trying the reusable "Diva menstrual cup" instead, which doesn't make me very confident at the beach. But to my surprise, there is no period. Since my D&C procedure, my period cycles have been shorter rather than longer, hence the surprise. I don't expect to get pregnant on the first try, so I decide to enjoy my beach party.

Another week goes by and still no bleeding. My girlfriend from New York calls me and announces she's finally pregnant at 38. She's happy although she's been feeling really lousy, suffering from a lack of sleep, unbearable constipation, and endless fatigue. "I really feel with you, girl, but it will pass in a few weeks, just be patient," I say trying to comfort her.

The next day I notice that my very regular stool is playing tricks on me. Normally, I go right after a few sips of my morning coffee or right after my healthy breakfast (consisting of homemade granola, plain yogurt and fresh fruit, pretty much every single day), but this time, nothing. Hmm. Over the next few days, I experience difficulties staying asleep, waking up around

3 am, and not being able to go back to my deep sleep. That's new too. By the end of the week, my husband asks about my period, and I start considering the option of actually being pregnant. But I'm in no rush to get a pregnancy test. I guess I don't want to get overexcited. By the time I buy a home pregnancy test, 2 weeks after my expected period, I'm quite sure it will be positive. And the indicator turns positive in a few seconds.

"We must have been bunnies in the past life," my husband reacts with a smirk. "We already got pregnant twice on the first try; that doesn't happen too often at our age." I have to admit: my nerdy scientist husband is actually funny, sometimes!

Chapter 30: I Hate Being Pregnant

Now that I'm pregnant, again, I want to do everything I can to prevent another miscarriage; meaning any aspect I can make a difference on. This time: no wine, no hard work around the house and garden, and lots of rest. Well, some things are easier said than done. Alcohol—not a problem. All the other "no's" —I'll try my best.

The following weeks are everything but enjoyable. My morning sickness (I have not experienced in my previous two pregnancies) has been lasting the whole day. Thankfully, I haven't vomited once, but my overall fatigue, nausea, and headaches, resulting mainly from a lack of sleep, have really caught up with me. I feel like a walking zombie. I have lost some weight, which is not necessarily a bad thing, but given the fact that I'm normally about 127 pounds at 5'-9" tall, losing weight in this condition is not quite desirable.

My appetite has been funky too. I'm a total foodie. I love to cook and experiment with dishes, but this time I'm completely turned off by any food or even the idea of eating. Not that I don't eat, but my desire for food has disappeared. I still consume about the same amounts as before; however, the joy is not quite there. That's very frustrating for me, as I'm the main food supplier and chef du casa.

I'm about 8 weeks pregnant now, and I just decided it's time for my blood work to be done to confirm my new condition. Since I don't have a doctor, once again, I ask my general doctor and friend to give me all the necessary referrals. Funny enough, she already knew about my recent miscarriage from my husband who saw her recently, and she's extremely supportive and happy I got pregnant so fast.

"This time everything will work out for you, I know it!" she tells me with a huge smile on the way out.

Positive encouragement always helps, although I know deep down that she can't influence any of it. But still better than my last gynecologist who was quick to remind me that "Yes, it (another miscarriage) can happen again," right on my first visit after my D&C. And yes, that's one of the reasons I decided not to use him for another pregnancy. The other reason was that his office has a "patient selection process," which I was aware of since I had to go through it before becoming his patient. What I wasn't aware of is that although I was already his patient, with each new pregnancy he would "evaluate me" and decide whether he wants to be my doctor or not. Well, that was enough for me to officially drop him as my doctor.

As we say in Czech, "That coffee was just too strong for me."

This time, my blood and urine results arrive only 3 days later, confirming my pregnancy.

Chapter 31: What To Do with a Horny Husband When You Are Feeling Sick

As we say in Czech, "There are two kinds of men: the smart ones and the married ones."

Men are just a different species altogether; so don't beat yourself if you feel like you are not "normal" right now [being pregnant]. Men can never understand the physical, psychological, or emotional condition women experience every month, during pregnancy, during childbirth, or recovering from delivery. Some men might be more understanding and caring, but most can't help but focus on their own needs. Unless you are literally dropping on your face and crying a river, they think you are just being dramatic. That's the way nature designed us. I wouldn't even bother trying to change that. Maybe finding a way to get what you want in the relationship could compensate for all the pain.

And when it comes to sex, it's the same story. I spoke to several women who either considered themselves obsessed with sex (nymphomaniacs) or had a real physical need for it every day, and most of them agreed that there were times both during pregnancy and after delivery when the idea of sex was actually making them sick.

So what shall we do with a horny husband when we feel like s..t? Unfortunately, men have two heads and sometimes they use the wrong one to make real-time decisions. And although women only have one head, by nature they are designed to use it wisely. So whatever you decide, make sure you don't offend your husband, but at the same time don't make yourself do things you are not fit for.

Chapter 32: Morning Boost with Lemon Water

Although I can't complain about having severe morning sickness—I haven't vomited once so far—my nausea and dizziness do last for most of the day. Plus my energy level is close to zero, making it hard to cope with my over-energetic now 4-year old monkey. A friend, who recently dealt with severe gastrointestinal issues and experienced weakness and loss of energy and appetite, recommended a morning glass of lemon water to help me better cope with my new condition.

The benefits of lemon/lime water are nothing new and I always liked the taste. I guess we all get a bit lazy once consumed by our daily routines so even the idea of squeezing a lemon into a glass of water might seem like a huge effort sometimes. Yet, I made a commitment to try it out.

After a little bit of research, I became even more encouraged since the number of benefits outweighed my humble expectations. Mainly, the improvement of digestion and boost to the immune system won me over. Although my constipation has gotten better (courtesy of papaya fruit), not only do my excessive gassiness and bloatedness often keep me from sleeping, they also make me feel uncomfortable around other people.

Another important quality of lemon water is the boost of energy, especially first thing in the morning. Although I've been practicing my morning yoga routine every single day, and that really helps my aching body to wake up, it doesn't always give me a boost of energy. Lemon/lime water supposedly will.

Other benefits, such as cleansing the body from toxins, alkalizing our over-acidified body, hydration, or reducing inflammation, are all very needed qualities right now. There is really nothing to lose trying it out.

After 1 week of drinking a glass of room-temperature lemon water first thing in the morning, and sometimes a few times a day, I have to attest that I do feel better. Although my skeptic husband notes, "It's all in my head," as long as I feel better knowing I'm doing something good for my body too, I really don't care what he says. After all, he has no idea how I truly feel.

Today he asked me why I'm in such a bad mood. "Bad mood?" I reply. "I'm not in a bad mood, I just feel like sh..t, that's all. Thanks for asking!"

Chapter 33: Time for Sono

As I'm approaching the end of my 8th week, I realize it might be time to get my first sonogram done to make sure my pregnancy is going well. Since I still don't have a gynecologist selected, I ask my general doctor to give me another referral. And while I'm at her office, she also reviews the results of my blood and urine tests and confirms that everything looks good. I specifically ask about my HCG quantitative levels, which I was monitoring closely during my previous pregnancy that ended in miscarriage. I bring my lab results from the previous pregnancy along with the new ones since the values are very different. While my previous pregnancy showed a value of 20,487, my current pregnancy showed a value of 106,300, both corresponding to about 8 weeks of gestational age. Naturally, such a huge difference caught my attention, even though according to the American Pregnancy Association the expected value for 7–8 weeks can range from 7,650 to 229,000 mIU/ml. My general doctor agrees and assures me that the current value looks more appropriate. She's a bit surprised that my previous gynecologist wasn't concerned with such a low value, as that could have already been a sign of improper fetal development.

Oh well, it is what it is. Another reason I should never go back to him. It's time to move forward, so I ask her to recommend a good gynecologist, preferably nearby, so I don't have to commute. She recommends two doctors who she works with at the hospital (1 day a week, she also works at the pediatric ER). Although one is a female and the other is male, and I'm ready for a female doctor, my general doctor favors the male doctor. He's younger than most doctors around here, in his late 30s, and therefore he's more open-minded and easy to talk to, according to her. We shall see then.

Chapter 34: Doctors, Oh Doctors

As we say in Czech,

"Six of one, half a dozen of the other."

I don't have many expectations, but I also don't have many choices at this point. I'm almost 10 weeks pregnant, and most doctors will not accept new patients at this stage anymore. Today is the day I'm going to check out these two doctors, who both happened to have their offices at the hospital where I previously gave birth, so I feel a certain level of comfort.

Despite my general doctor's preference for the younger male doctor, I walk into the office of the older female doctor first and ask the receptionist if they accept new patients. She asks for the date of my last menstruation, then checks her calendar, and within few seconds she shakes her head.

"Unfortunately, in April we are already overbooked, so the doctor would not be able to take you in."

Alright, that was quick. But she points me to the other doctor's office, which is literally next door. As I'm walking out, I realize that the waiting room is completely packed to the ceiling. So, maybe it's a good thing they didn't accept me, as I would be spending my precious free time waiting in this crowded room. And as I'm walking into the other doctor's office, I'm surprised by the relatively empty waiting room. That's a nice change, but it does make me wonder how good this other doctor is. I ask the receptionist if they accept new pregnant patients, and she replies that they do, but I would have to come back on Friday, since that's the day the doctor "interviews" new patients. She's all smiles, so I smile back, thank her, and respond that I'll be back on Friday then.

Chapter 35: The New Doctor

A few days later, on Friday morning, I arrive at the new prospective doctor's office early so I don't have to camp out there all day. The waiting room is completely empty, and another nurse-receptionist arrives just a few minutes after me. She asks me what I'm waiting for, then hands me a writing pad with several papers to fill out and requests my insurance card and identification.

Ten minutes later, she informs me that the doctor is upstairs in the delivery room, but he could see me in about half an hour, if that's ok with me.

"That's totally fine with me, thank you, I can wait for him here, no problem." She gives me a smile and goes back to her paperwork.

People start arriving. First, a woman about my age, with a daughter who looks 13 or 14, and the daughter's boyfriend. I overhear her mom talking to the nurse, saying it's her daughter's first pregnancy, she's 4 weeks pregnant, and they are all very excited. A few more women enter the room, then another mom with a teenage daughter. The first mom-daughter pair go in before me for an interview. Then a doctor rushes in, and the nurse calls me right in.

"Good morning, so what can I do for you?" the doctor asks before looking at my newly created record file.

"Well, I'm about 9 weeks pregnant, looking for a new doctor, and you came highly recommended by my general doctor, Kristina," I reply back. The rest of the conversation is rather pleasant; we discuss all my previous issues and non-issues, and of course my preferences for birth. Then comes the genetic testing topic, which, at my age, is a big factor in a healthy pregnancy, as I mentioned before. The doctor strongly suggests considering amniocentesis, as it's the only test that is diagnostic (as opposed to screening) and about 99% accurate. I tell him I didn't do "amnio" with my first child; I refused it because of the possible risk of pregnancy complications or miscarriage, and my previous doctor didn't insist on it, as everything else looked normal. I explain that I would prefer to start with the first and second trimester combined screenings, and based on the results I would decide further. Although he doesn't appear super content with my plan, he doesn't push the subject anymore.

"Alright then. So shall we take a look at the baby now? I understand this will be your first sonogram, correct?"

"Yes, that's correct," I reply. In the exam room I start feeling a bit anxious. It reminds me of the last sonogram exam I had about 6 months ago, which brought back memories about my previous pregnancy. But I take a deep breath and try to relax. As the doctor searches for the fetus in my uterus, I follow the monitor, trying to determine what I'm looking at. He doesn't say a word until we see the baby and it appears to be moving. I must admit I feel instant relief.

"Well, here is our little one, and he seems to be doing fine." About a minute later, the doctor adds: "You seem to be quite an educated and sophisticated woman, so I'll be very open with you. I already see something that worries me a bit." Then he points to a round mass of something that's about the size of the baby's head.

"What is it?" I ask.

"It appears to be the intestines, which by now should be mostly inside the baby's belly. What worries me is the size of it, and at this point I can't quite tell if that mass includes only the intestines or other organs too. Therefore, I would like you to see a perinatal specialist, who has better equipment than I do and can determine what exactly we are looking at and what are the possible risks, if any."

Then his nurse enters telling him that he needs to return back to the delivery room. "If you can wait about an hour, I can explain the condition and its risks in more details."

"I'll wait," I reply, pretty calmly.

"Why don't you get a cup of coffee in the meantime? Or if you want, call your husband and look up these two conditions." He writes *Omphalocele*[15] and *Gastroschisis*[16] on a piece of paper and then rushes out

---

[15] Omphalocele is a rare abdominal wall defect in which the intestines, liver, and occasionally other organs remain outside of the abdomen in a sac because of a defect in the development of the muscles of the abdominal wall. It occurs in 1/4,000 births and is associated with a high rate of mortality (25%) and severe malformations, such as cardiac anomalies (50%) and neural tube defects (40%). Approximately 15% of live-born infants with omphalocele have chromosomal abnormalities.

[16] Gastroschisis is a birth defect of the abdominal wall. The baby's intestines stick outside of the baby's body,

of the room.

I call my husband and explain what the doctor has found and his possible concerns. My husband being a scientific nerd and a skeptic, not trusting any doctor, looks up the conditions in relation to the gestational age and assures me that at 9 weeks it's still very common that the intestines are outside the baby's belly. Also, research[17] shows that there's no way to diagnose omphalocele before week 11; hence, going to a specialist at this point would be a waste of time. So we should not stress ourselves out at this point.

As calm as I was before, this new possible finding—whether it's omphalocele or gastroschisis[18]—has made me super upset and freaked out too. Despite my husband's calming comments, my mind is all over the place.

---

through a hole beside the belly button. The hole can be small or large and sometimes other organs, such as the stomach and liver, can also stick outside of the baby's body.

[17] Fetal Omphalocele Detected Early in Pregnancy: Associated Anomalies and Outcomes

[18] Increasing Prevalence of Gastroschisis-14 States

When the doctor returns, he explains things once again, now in more detail, and insists I go to see the perinatal specialist as soon as possible. Being that it's Friday afternoon, and he can't get a hold of him over the phone, he recommends I make an appointment first thing Monday morning and return to see him right after that visit. On my way out the doctor tells me with a smile:

"Listen, I want you not to worry; let's take things one step at a time, and not jump to conclusions."

Thanks a lot, a-hole, I think to myself.

Chapter 36: Prepare a New Strategy

On the way home, I can't hold it in anymore, and I start crying. Then the first thing I do when I return home is research both conditions online, including visuals. That's a major mistake. My husband turns me away from the computer and calms me down:

"Look, based on what I've found, there's no reason to be concerned right now. One, it's quite common for intestines to stick out at 9 weeks and it should correct itself in the next week or so. And two, we don't quite know what he saw on the sonogram and neither does he. Rushing to a specialist just a few days after will not give us any answers either; it's too early to diagnose omphalocele or gastroschisis. What I think we should do is wait a week and instead of going to the specialist, get another opinion."

I recall I still have a valid referral from my general doctor for a sonogram. "Why don't we go to another sonogram place in about a week and see what they have to say without telling them what my doctor suspects?" I suggest.

My husband agrees that's a wise option. Good, now that we have a game plan I need to calm myself down and stop thinking about it. Although I originally planned on avoiding alcohol during this pregnancy, I feel that one glass of my favorite Shiraz would only do me good today.

Chapter 37: A Week Later Makes a Huge Difference

The following Friday, exactly 1 week after my first visit, I go to my favorite sonogram lab using my old referral. My husband joins me this time, just in case the news is not good, or in case there's a need to immediately double check what the sonogram technician finds.

The female technician is almost my friend now; she remembered my very first pregnancy—she was the one who confirmed my miscarriage only 6 months earlier, and now she will be delivering another important piece of information. My husband and I agree that we will not tell her about what my doctor was suspecting a week earlier, and we'll see what she finds and how she puts it. She's very professional and thorough, and a very pleasant lady, so the visit itself relaxes me despite my anxiety. About 20 minutes into the examination, she looks very content and assures me that we have a very healthy baby. My husband finally asks her if she can see anything of a concern, especially with the baby's intestines or other organs. She confirms they are almost entirely inside the belly cavity now, which corresponds to the gestational age, and she doesn't see one thing that we should be worried about. As a typical nerd, my husband keeps asking more questions and basically interviews her about her experience with abnormal cases and such.

We both leave with smiles on our faces after about 45 minutes, relieved and excited. As I'm leaving full of sunshine I don't even notice there is an old friend sitting in the waiting room, waving at me.

Chapter 38: Genetic Testing

I think it's time I reveal one of the reasons for my frustrations with the doctors and the medical system. After spending the first 20 years of my life in Europe, then about 15 years in the U.S. —but primarily in New York City—I now live in Puerto Rico. And as much as I love this island and enjoy my life in paradise, my recent frustrations are really making me bitter.

As a writer for a health and wellness publication (Living Green with Baby), I come across the latest research and health news every single day, so I consider myself quite informed about what's possible these days and what's not. Before I became pregnant a second time, in late 2013, I learned about a new study from England that confirmed that routine screening during the first trimester using a non-invasive blood test that analyzes fetal DNA can accurately detect Down syndrome and other genetic fetal abnormalities. That made me very happy since this new finding could replace the currently available screening strategies, such as Chorionic villus sampling (CVS) and amniocentesis, both posing a risk of miscarriage or damage to the fetus. Although I was over 35 with my first pregnancy in 2010, I declined undergoing either of these invasive tests, mainly due to the risk. My blood tests were indicating either no or really low risk of genetic abnormalities, so my husband and I found it absolutely unnecessary.

However, now I'm 41 and really want to take advantage of this new screening test, sometimes referred to as *MaterniT21*. When I ask my doctor about it, he has no problem writing me a referral for the lab. Once I bring it to the lab, they look at me like I just returned from Mars. They have never heard about this type of blood test, let alone were they able to find the relevant insurance code for it. My lab technician interviews me about it, then calls my insurance, but can't get one straight answer. That really confuses me since this test has already been around for several years worldwide, and Puerto Rico has a comparable healthcare system to the mainland U.S. A few days later, I receive a call from my lab technician informing me that the first portion of the test could be done in Puerto Rico but is only partially covered by the insurance and my co-pay would be about $500. Wow. But here comes the big BUT. The second part of the test, which is essential for the screening results, can't be done locally; it would have to be shipped to California and would cost me about $2,000. Or, they can ship my blood samples there for the complete analysis, which will cost me only $5,000 total. Had I known that before, I would have flown to New York and had it done there. It's too late now, so my only option is to continue with my other prenatal screenings and go from there. If I have to go through amniocentesis this time, then so be it.

As I'm working on updates and revisions of this book for its second edition, a friend of mine who is currently pregnant at 40 with her first child, informs me about another new non-invasive prenatal testing based on cell-free DNA analysis called the Harmony Prenatal Test. This screening test can be performed as early as week 10 of pregnancy. Also, it's more accurate than traditional Down syndrome blood tests since it's much less likely to give a false-positive result compared to traditional tests such as the first trimester screening test. That means, that your doctor would less likely recommend a follow-up diagnostic testing, such as amniocentesis.

Harmony also tests for two other genetic conditions, trisomy 18 (Edward syndrome) and trisomy 13 (Patau syndrome), and you have an option to evaluate fetal sex, X and Y sex chromosomes.

According to a large, multicenter cohort study published in April 2015 in the New England Journal of Medicine[19], researches found that cfDNA testing had a higher sensitivity and specificity than did standard screening for the detection of trisomy 21 in a general prenatal-screening population. The false positive rate of cfDNA testing was nearly 100 times lower than that of standard screening. Their study included pregnant women of all risk levels, and 76% were under the age of 35 years. They found that cfDNA testing was more sensitive than standard screening and yielded lower false positive rates, regardless of maternal age.

Thanks to ongoing research, pregnant women will keep having more options to avoid invasive diagnostic tests such as CVS and amniocentesis. This is all great news, since no expectant parent, especially not after 40, wants to expose their baby to a risky procedure.

---

[19] Cell-free DNA Analysis for Noninvasive Examination of Trisomy

Chapter 39: Pregnancy and Religion

With all due respect to people of religion, being pregnant in a highly religious country makes me feel like I'm constantly walking on eggshells.

When I first met my current gynecologist, I wasn't quite sure how to approach certain questions, not knowing his religious status and his take on abortion. Thankfully, he asked about my position on pregnancy termination first, just in case my genetic tests would indicate some problems or complications. That question made me feel very at ease with him. I explained that I grew up in an atheist environment, I'm a total pragmatist, plus I'm married to a scientist who, although he's of Puerto Rican descent, is also an atheist. With that said, neither me nor my husband would want to continue a pregnancy that would lead to an unhealthy, disabled, or otherwise compromised human being. We believe in quality of life, and wouldn't put a child through a difficult childhood and adulthood with physical and/or health complications caused by genetic abnormalities. My gynecologist fully agreed with me on that subject and explained that the abortion rate is currently actually pretty high. That statement shocked me. I guess I always assumed that most religious people would not choose to terminate pregnancies. He added that actually it's often young and very religious women (even girls) who come to him to abort their otherwise healthy pregnancies to avoid shame from their churches, families, or communities. What a sad reality!

When discussing the subject with my husband, we found that abortion data can be hard to come by anywhere, not just for the U.S. territory. Nevertheless, my husband wasn't completely surprised. He recalled many years ago going out with a local girl once who was pressured by her parents to sew back her hymen after losing her virginity to a boyfriend. And she did.

Chapter 40: Stress is Worse Than Any Other Health Condition

As we say in Czech, "A happy mind makes for half of your good health."

We all know stress is bad for us. And particularly during pregnancy, we should keep our calm. But how can you "keep your calm" when you are constantly dealing with uncertain situations and waiting periods that only contribute to anxiety and additional stress? I personally don't believe a "stress-less" pregnancy is possible. Even though my first pregnancy was relatively easy, just waiting for test results or sometimes even for the doctor's appointment wasn't easy at all. Especially today, with fast and easy access to information online, we can get overwhelmed with all sorts of data and worry about possible outcomes that might not even concern us.

Stress can be really damaging, especially to the expectant mom. If our stress goes untreated or without relief, it can lead to a condition called *distress* (a negative stress reaction). Distress can then cause physical symptoms such as high blood pressure, migraines, chest pain, insomnia, digestive issues and others. Although I consider myself a relatively calm person, I have experienced some of the above symptoms myself. Some scientific research also suggests that stress can cause or exacerbate certain symptoms and even diseases.

Here are some scary facts (via WebMD):

- *43% of all adults suffer harmful health effects from stress;*
- *75–90% of all doctor's office visits are for stress-related illnesses and complaints;*
- *Stress can play a part in problems such as headaches, high blood pressure, heart problems, diabetes, skin conditions, asthma, arthritis, depression, and anxiety;*
- *The Occupational Safety and Health Administration (OSHA) declared stress a hazard of the workplace. Stress costs American industry more than $300 billion each year;*

- *The lifetime prevalence of an emotional disorder is more than 50%, and often due to chronic, untreated stress reactions.*

Those are some serious numbers. As numerous studies suggest[20], if you are pregnant and your stress becomes constant, the effects on you and your baby could be lasting. Here is what is happening physically and psychologically to your body (via WebMD): "*When you're stressed, your body goes into "fight or flight" mode, releasing a burst of cortisol and other stress hormones. These are the same hormones that rise when you are in danger. They prepare you to run by sending a blast of fuel to your muscles and making your heart pump faster. Therefore, it's really critical to pay attention to any persisting stress and to deal with it. Once you deal with it, your stress response will diminish and your body can go back into its balance.*"

As Susan Andrews, PhD, a clinical neuropsychologist and author of the book *Stress*

---

[20] Prenatal maternal stress: effects on pregnancy and the (unborn) child

Stress during pregnancy is associated with developmental outcome in infancy

Psychosocial stress in pregnancy and its relation to low birth weight

Solutions for Pregnant Moms: How Breaking Free From Stress Can Boost Your Baby's Potential explains: "The kind of stress that's really damaging is the kind that doesn't let up. In fact, constant stress could alter your body's stress management system, causing it to overreact and trigger an inflammatory response."

Maternal inflammation has then been linked not only to poorer pregnancy health (possibly causing Polycystic ovary syndrome[21] and other health complications), but also to developmental problems in babies that could lead to serious disorders, including schizophrenia[22]or autism[23].

There you have it! So the question is: What actually carries a higher risk for us, pregnant moms, and our babies? Doing every single test that's available (as some moms-to-be do these days) just to make sure we don't miss anything important, while risking a miscarriage or other possible health consequence and

---

[21] Low-Grade Chronic Inflammation in Pregnant Women With Polycystic Ovary Syndrome

[22] Inflammation in Pregnancy Strongly Linked to Schizophrenia

[23] Brain's Inflammatory Response in Overdrive May Contribute to Common Brain Disorders

then stressing and worrying about the results? Or finding a balance among all the craziness, choosing the right counselors you fully trust, making your own decisions, and learning to relax as much as possible? Knowing now what a constant stress can do, I go with selecting wisely, following my gut feeling, and going with what I find necessary for a given situation; of course after consulting with my doctor and my husband, since we are in this together 50-50.

I have a long way to go learning how to cope with stressful decisions and situations, but today I learned to accept my own decision once I make it.

Chapter 41: Peace of Mind

Today is my first check-up after all the stress of genetic testing. My doctor notes I have only gained 8 pounds in my pregnancy so far, but given my active life and good health, he's not worried. I'm definitely not concerned since I only gained 15 pounds during my first pregnancy. And although my previous gynecologist was very concerned that my boy will be a small baby, my Czech gynecologist I consulted with via email assured me that my baby will catch up in no time. And he sure did. Now that all the stress is over and I didn't have to go through amniocentesis, I feel like I should allow myself a glass of red wine once a week. A small glass after dinner helps me relax both my mind and my body, and I sleep like a baby myself.

Chapter 42: Week 24

I know it's the holidays and I've been attending parties, therefore eating more sweets and more food than I normally do, but I'm also more active since my boy is out of school and I'm trying to finish up an almost-completed project. I feel I'm more on my feet than ever before, yet my belly feels like it has just exploded. Last night I weighed myself for the first time since my last doctor's visit 2 weeks ago, and it looks like I gained 13 pounds since the beginning of my pregnancy, which means I gained 5 pounds during the last two weeks alone. For better or worse, I don't feel or look like a "cow," but the sudden gain causes quite a discomfort and pressure in my abdominal area. Thanks to my regular stretching and yoga twice a day, I don't have any back pain so far, but my varicose veins are popping out and even hurt to touch.

After my first pregnancy I didn't have any stretch marks, partially thanks to all those yoga stretches, and also thanks to literally buttering my belly before bedtime with a secret lotion my good friend prepared just for me. The "secret" is actually nothing new, the mixture contained unrefined Shea butter, bee wax, extra virgin olive and coconut oils, Vitamin E, and some other essential oils. This time I'm doing it again—it's a simple remedy that makes my aching body feel better and it works on my skin too.

Chapter 43: Severe Muscle Spasms

A brand new phenomenon I didn't experience during my previous pregnancies has appeared out of the blue. As I twist and turn a lot during the night, my body tends to stretch while changing positions, causing muscle cramps or even spasms. Of course they are quite common during pregnancy; however, my spasms have started intensifying and are sometimes so severe that the muscle pain remains even throughout the day. They usually occur during the early morning hours; so far I haven't experienced them later in the day. My chiropractor suggests that such severe spasms might have caused micro tears in my muscle tissue similar to sport injuries; therefore, the pain will continue until the muscle heals properly.

When I consult my gynecologist, the first thing he asks is if I take enough calcium and magnesium. I assure him that on top of my prenatal vitamin, I take a calcium supplements before bedtime, and I consume ample amount of foods high in calcium including dairy, nuts, seeds, dark leafy veggies, broccoli, beans, and oranges on a daily basis. Plus, I regularly practice yoga and stretching throughout the day.

"That's pretty unusual, I have to say," he replies. "You are doing everything right, definitely more than an average expectant mama, so what I would recommend to try out is to do absolutely nothing for about 3 days. And I mean nothing, including yoga, other exercise, or any physical activity. It's possible your body is so exhausted that all it needs is a real rest."

Well, that's easy to say, but the reality of everyday life is different. First, I can't imagine myself lying down and resting for 3 days even if I could afford such a luxury. Second, I can't afford such a luxury, period. Plus stretching every morning, especially after a rough night, helps me become functional again instead of being a zombie all day. But I'll do my best with daily resting time.

As the weeks go by, the spasms do slowly mellow down and become rather rare. But even at week 35, I still experience them some nights. They haven't been as severe as before, but then again, my whole body is so tired these days that I wouldn't be able to tell if my legs hurt because of night spasms, lack of sleep, or carrying the excessive weight.

Chapter 44: Manual Labor During Pregnancy

As we say in Czech, "The devil never sleeps."

Timing is never perfect, and sometimes it happens that we get more work than we wish for when we need it the least. It just so happened that when I was pregnant with my first child 5 years ago, we had just purchased a house, and being an architect and a perfectionist, I couldn't help myself and had to do a full "gut-rehab" renovation before moving in, starting about a month after my son was born. Although the final result was quite exceptional, I almost "killed myself" managing the whole show while caring for a newborn and my weight went down to 119 pounds (which is way below my normal weight).

Well, the devil never sleeps and now, right around the time of my current pregnancy, we have a unique opportunity to acquire an investment property. Being *me*, I decide to do another full "gut-rehab" renovation. This time, I think to myself, it will be much easier, as now I can speak Spanish and know local contractors and their ways. Well, as it happens, it's not any easier at all. I've been working full time for about 4 months straight; fulfilling the roles of the architect, supplier, project manager, and investor in one. Moreover, the last 2 weeks before our first tenants are supposed to move in, I have to perform all sorts of manual labor myself since my contractor is officially finished. Although I'm being extremely careful, I end up drilling close to 100 holes in rigid concrete, painting some wood, walls, and even refinishing concrete countertops. I avoid using any harmful or toxic materials and always wear protective clothing and a mask; however, the intensity of this labor is almost exceeding my physical abilities at this time. I'm surprised myself I haven't gotten sick from the exhaustion yet.

Today is the official last day of my work, and all I have to do is install a relatively lightweight wire mesh shelf in a closet. It's an easy task until my leveling tool falls out of my clumsy hand, and in an attempt to catch it so it doesn't break, the shelf gets loose and falls on top of my foot. And since this is one of the last things I have to do before going home, I'm not even wearing proper footwear. As the shelf hits the floor after falling down from about 5-foot height its wire hits my flesh. I can't even describe the excruciating pain I feel right now. I'm literally speechless. I sit down on the floor with my leg extended and watch it turn yellow and blue and swollen while crying and cussing aloud. But I have no other choice than to get myself together. I rub some alcohol on the area, and then I get the job done. The injury turns out to be very mild with my foot just severely bruised, but it takes about 4 weeks before the area is completely healed. And even after 2 months, I still can't bend my foot for yoga like I used to. I'm sure pregnancy has something to do with the body's ability to recover.

In the end, everybody loves the house, so I guess it wasn't all just wasted time and energy on my part.

My mom keeps reminding me that she doesn't want to hear me complaining if the little one turns out to be hyperactive or sensitive to noise since I have caused it myself with all this unnecessary work. I guess we just have to wait and see. And although I wouldn't recommend doing such crazy things to any expectant mama, knowing myself, I would probably do it again.

Chapter 45: Measles Outbreak

The recent measles outbreak in California has created a lot of buzz all over, including my green parenting website. Although I can sympathize with some parents who have to deal with their child's adverse reaction to a vaccine (our boy has recently experienced moderate swelling after the DTaP vaccine and was even sent home from school claiming he might have *cellulitis* infection), anti-vaccine statements really get to me, especially at a time of an unnecessary outbreak. I'm way beyond the point of having discussions with my anti-vaccine friends about what "the real truth" is. Similarly, like I don't discuss religion, I refuse to argue about facts that are ignored even by many educated and sophisticated people. It's upsetting and sad. I've been trying to ignore all the comments and silly memes in social media making fun of the outbreak, such as "If I hear measles one more time, I will….." It's childish, in my opinion.

However, today a whole new discussion got stirred up on my website on the subject, after one "Alternative mama" posts: "Don't let the vaccine

Gestapo get you!!! Measles isn't that big of a deal!" Such statement makes me quite angry, as it's in response to an article I re-posted as information to parents outlining 9 facts everybody should know about measles. And right in the opening paragraph, it states, "*It's the most infectious disease known to humanity, even more infectious than Ebola or SARS.*" How can anybody question such a fact is beyond me. Her comment opens up such a heated discussion with other followers that this "poor alternative mama" has no chance of arguing her blurb and doesn't even attempt to respond in the end.

But the situation is concerning, as the outbreak is spreading, and I do have a 4-year old who is surrounded by kids of such "alternative mamas"—plus I'm currently pregnant. So what happens if the outbreak reaches my town or community? Do I stay locked up in the house just to protect my newborn child and myself? It's a shame that people like me have to be afraid to leave the house not to get exposed to potentially dangerous viruses just because some individuals don't believe in scientific facts. While we live in a world with progressive medicine where infectious diseases have almost been eradicated.

Then I come across an article titled *I'm Autistic, And Believe Me, It's A Lot Better Than Measles,*[24] where an adult woman describes her personal experience of suffering from severe measles and compares it to her life as someone with autism. Definitely a good read that puts this disease [measles] into perspective.

Since the subject of vaccinations is so confusing to many people, my husband has researched and compiled data currently available from verified and respected medical and scientific sources into an article called *A Parents' Guide to Children's Vaccinations*, which I'm including at the end of this book as a resource and reference for future moms.

---

[24] I'm Autistic, And Believe Me, It's A Lot Better Than Measles

Chapter 46: Vaccines and Pregnancy

No doctor has ever asked about my vaccination history before conception, but in light of the recent measles outbreak, I do my homework about what's recommended and what's not. Those of us who were vaccinated with MMR vaccine as children should still have antibodies that will protect our babies during pregnancy and a few months after they're born[25]. This gets confirmed with a simple blood test for Rubella. For women who are planning pregnancy and are possibly exposed to the virus, CDC recommends getting a boost at least 4 weeks before conception. There are certain vaccines recommended for all adults to keep on schedule, such as Tetanus and Hepatitis A and B, which can be obtained during pregnancy as well, if necessary. Others are recommended postpartum.

Based on my medical history and current health

---

[25] Immunology 101 Series: To Keep You and Your Baby Safe, Vaccines Are Expected When You're Expecting

Vaccines for pregnant women

condition, my doctor doesn't think it's necessary to provide any boosts or additional vaccinations. However, he does recommend staying away from busy public spaces like shopping centers or big events, especially during weekends and the holidays, to avoid exposure and limit my possible risk of contracting viruses and diseases. So I do.

Chapter 47: Delivery Options and Age

Many of my friends and acquaintances have been asking me about how I'm going to deliver the baby. Honestly, I'm not going to play a hero this time. Not that I was a hero the first time around, but I wanted a natural childbirth, if possible, and I got it. This time I'm a bit older, and over 40, so I'd rather play it safe. I would not consider a homebirth, but if a natural delivery is possible, I would prefer it. I'm not opposing any medication either. If a C-section will be necessary due to my health situation or an emergency, I would not hesitate a minute, but it would definitely not be my first choice.

Talking about C-sections[26], new research from the University College Cork in Ireland indicates that babies born via C-section could be at a 21% greater risk of developing an autism spectrum disorder (ASD).

---

[26] Association Between Obstetric Mode of Delivery and Autism Spectrum Disorder

Chapter 48: Preterm Delivery

My first son was born unexpectedly and spontaneously at 38 weeks, and I guess I have always assumed it would be the same with the second baby as well. But nothing is ever guaranteed. Since I'm 41 now, my doctor informs me that the risk of birth complications and/or stillbirth past 38 weeks of pregnancy double for women my age, and he would prefer I not carry beyond week 39. What does that mean, exactly? The risk of stillbirth is generally about 1 in 1,000, so in my case the risk increases to 2 in 1,000. Which, as my statistician husband puts it, is still very unlikely. But, neither my husband nor I are willing to take any risks, especially at the end of such a rocky road. We agree with my doctor that if labor doesn't come spontaneously by the end of the 39th week, we will schedule an induction.

Official figures show the following statistics: the older a woman is, the higher her risk for preterm delivery. Women over 35 are 20% more likely to deliver preterm. Of those born at 32 to 35 weeks gestation, 98% survive. Babies born at less than 28 weeks are at the highest risk for problems. Of those very preterm babies, 20 to 40% develop lasting disabilities. Infants born after 34 weeks, however, have excellent chances and only face possible learning or behavioral disabilities. Today, more than one in 10 babies born to mothers over the age of 40 is premature.

Chapter 49: Varicose Veins

Even though I have had varicose veins since my 20s, thanks to my genetic predisposition, each of my pregnancies brings it to another level. Yes, I know it's very common, and being on my feet most of the day doesn't help either, but it got to a point that my left leg (which has always been more susceptible to the problem) hurts so much, that I have to do something about it.

First, I try raising my leg on a pillow while sleeping, either during the day or at night. That helps relieve the pain a bit, but the veins continue appearing.

When I ask my doctor, he immediately recommends using special stockings that will restrict the blood flow in the area. I'm quite familiar with them, since my mom has been using them on her own varicose veins for decades. I also know that they shouldn't be used 24/7, especially not at night when the legs are in a horizontal position. However, I live in the tropics and the idea of wearing any kind of stockings during the day is almost unbearable. Maybe if I sat in an air-conditioned office all day this would be an option, but I don't. I do get myself something like a knee brace that also covers a significant area below my knee, and I do wear it during the day while on my feet. During the night, I raise my leg and use a cooling pad to reduce inflammation of the area. I think this combination does help with the pain, but the varicose veins do not disappear.

Chapter 50: Allergies

Child allergies, especially food allergies, are a serious problem these days. Based on data from the Food Allergy Research & Education (FARE) organization, today one in every 13 children has some kind of a food allergy. The number of allergic and asthmatic children multiplied 2 to 3 times during the last decades of the 20th century, and specifically food allergies continue to increase. According to Popular Science[27], today's children aren't spending enough time outdoors and aren't getting enough natural vitamin D, which supports their immune system. Since their natural immunity can't develop properly, their bodies aren't able to properly identify harmless substances and they overreact in form of allergic reaction. As Anne Muñoz-Furlong, CEO of the nonprofit Food Allergy and Anaphylaxis Network, noted: "*Scientific progress, including hygiene and successful treatments for infections, has left children's immune systems with little to do, so they go looking for things to attack. As Live Science puts it, they're bored*."

---

[27] Why Are so Many Kids Allergic to Peanuts
Peanut Allergy Cases Triple in 10 Years

Then there is also an exposure to allergens, such as nuts, during pregnancy. Not only do most nuts provide important nutrients to the pregnant mom and her unborn child, consuming nuts during pregnancy can also lower the child's chances of future food allergies, according to a 2014 study published in the journal JAMA Pediatrics[28]. Researchers at Harvard Medical School collected and analyzed data on more than 8,200 children and reported that women who ate nuts before, during and after their pregnancies—at least five times a week—had the lowest risk of their children developing a nut allergy.

That's definitely good news for me since I love eating nuts as fast snacks or on-the-go. My personal favorites are almonds, which contain good amounts of calcium and iron, both essential minerals for proper baby development as well as healthy fats. Eating nuts on a daily basis (and not only during pregnancy) can also help regulate weight gain. My only problem with hard nuts, such as almonds, is that I keep having dental "injuries," probably due to my current calcium depletion.

---

[28] Children at Lower Risk for Peanut, Tree Nut Allergies if Moms Ate More Nuts While Pregnant

I don't remember ever having as many dental issues in my life as I've had during these last two pregnancies. I guess another age factor. Of course, there are solutions to avoid any injuries, such as soaking them first in warm water to soften them up or consuming them in butter form. But I still prefer them in their natural raw form.

Chapter 51: Natural Ways to Induce Labor

With my first pregnancy, things went pretty fast. I think that a lot of laughing, dancing, and a legendary dark chocolate cake at my husband's birthday party the night before, really did the trick. But who really knows.

This time around, things are a bit different. Not only am I 5 years older, overworked, and therefore physically really tired, I'm also sort of over this pregnancy and hoping things will just go fast. At 37.5 weeks, my doctor tells me today that my baby has dropped significantly since the week before and he can now feel his head. My cervix is over 1 cm dilated and the labor is 75% effaced. So the process has started, and we can either wait or help it a bit. Of course, sex is always a good stimulant, and honestly, I have lately been quite for it, but usually early in the morning when my husband is surfing or early afternoon when my husband is working. There's always "Santa's little helper," as we call my favorite French toy, but that doesn't get the sperm to soften up the cervix. There's also the "convenience of timing" to consider. My husband is giving an important exam in two days so it would be rather inconvenient to go into labor before that. But right after that is over we can effectively work on it daily and see how the little one responds.

I have also just found out that certain tropical fruits, such as pineapple, mango, or papaya, contain an enzyme called *bromelain*, which is believed to help soften the cervix and stimulate labor. That's really good news for me since there's an abundance of these fruits where we live. I also happen to love papayas and have overproducing papaya plants in my own garden. Fresh papaya is part of my daily diet, and coincidentally I have been munching on cool papaya pieces (I keep them available in my fridge) every night to cool off from the tropical heat.

This weekend will mark the end of week 38, and our wedding anniversary will be 3 days later, so maybe those are all good reasons to get things pumping a bit. Chocolate cake is always welcome, although it's not officially supposed to bring on any contractions—at least it will make me happy and put me into mood. Oh, and I almost forgot that a good comedy has been doing me well too.

Well, I have a feeling this weekend we'll try to combine them all and see what happens.

Chapter 52: Giving Birth for the First Time

For my first baby, I was 38 weeks pregnant and on my weekly check-up my doctor told me that I'd been having contractions and that we would deliver my baby the following week, either naturally or with induction. I didn't quite understand what he meant, but since I didn't feel anything, I wasn't paying much attention to what he said. Technically, there's no such thing as having contractions for a week; there's pre-labor, which is different and can even last several weeks. So either this doctor didn't know what he was talking about, or he was attempting to conveniently schedule the delivery in his own itinerary.

It was Friday afternoon, and my girlfriends were throwing me a baby shower party on Saturday evening, so I had other things on my mind. To be honest, I really didn't want any baby shower because I hate being a center of attention. For the same reason, I never really have birthday parties either, and even refused to have a wedding party. But since my friends insisted and it happened to be my husband's birthday too, I agreed that we'd do a combined celebration to alleviate some of the pressure. I ordered a special dark chocolate and strawberry cake for the hubby, and since I was the only one in the whole house who wasn't drinking, I sure took advantage of all the great food and the cake too—to a point that I was having stomach and intestinal cramps by the end of the party. The whole night, I experienced indigestion pain and felt very uncomfortable. What was I thinking! In the morning—which was Sunday—I did my regular yoga and stretching exercises and it did make me feel better. But the cramps continued. My husband joked, that probably all the good food caused me to have contractions. But when the cramps continued and slightly intensified after lunch, he called his sister, who's a nurse with 5 kids of her own, to ask her opinion. She asked me a few questions such as how strong these cramps were and how frequent and where exactly I felt them. Then she gave me the good news that I was in labor. She suggested that I start monitoring contractions from that point on, and once they start coming about 5 minutes apart, I should head for the hospital. Holy s..t! We both exclaimed at the same time.

That's great; we were so not ready for this. Our

plan was to spend the following 2 weeks buying baby stuff and preparing for delivery, and now we might have just a few hours to get ready. Then we both started laughing. My husband didn't hesitate and started searching online for any useful videos and information preparing for labor since we had not taken a single class on delivering a baby. We spent about an hour watching Lamaze videos and all sorts of other childbirth practices and recommendations. It totally reminded me of a scene from the film *Matrix,* when Trinity urgently needs to fly a helicopter. The operator instantly uploads that information directly into her brain, and once she receives it she flies off. Since we don't live in the matrix, I'm just going to have to rely on what I was able to absorb on the fly and my own gut instincts.

And so they came—contractions about 5 minutes apart. My husband and I checked in at the hospital. I still wasn't dilated enough, so the doctor had not yet arrived. Surprisingly, the pain felt quite manageable. It kind of reminded me of my constipation problems when I was about 8 years old. I also think that my yoga experience helped me with my breathing, which kept the pain to a minimum. The doctor arrived 3 hours after I checked into the hospital. He was dressed the way one would think someone would be dressed on a Sunday afternoon, with an orange polo shirt and beige slacks, as though he had come straight from the golf course, and I'm pretty sure he did. The pain of course was a bit stronger by then, but still not as bad as I had imagined. After filling out some paperwork, the doctor came back to my room and said,

"Okay, let's deliver the baby, shall we?"

I was taken to a different room, and placed on the delivery table. The doctor reminded me that he would ask me to push and when he did, I should take a deep breath and push while exhaling. We then continued doing this every 1 or 2 minutes.

Twenty minutes into the delivery, the doctor leaned toward my husband and said, "I'm very concerned since she's not pushing hard enough. I know she is older and tired, but taking too long could be damaging to the baby and to her too. I suggest I assist her through the use of a suction cup."

Since I was focusing on managing the pain and pushing, I didn't hear any of this. Then all of the sudden, I felt an excruciating pain. That must have been when the baby's head crowned a little after the doctor had inserted the suction cup in me. Of the entire delivery process for my first child, it was at that very moment that I recall feeling the most pain. Having said that, at least it didn't last long, and after a few seconds, the doctor handed me my baby. I recall my baby boy having a cone shaped head, sort like the Alien movies. But because of the whole ordeal, I didn't give it too much thought. It was only later that my husband told me that he freaked out when the doctor pulled out the baby with a very deformed head: "What happened to our baby?" He later realized that it was because of the suction cup, and after a few minutes, the head was already becoming rounder.

In the end, everything turned out ok with our first son. Although he had a bruised head for two weeks, nowadays he's a healthy, smart, extremely hyperactive boy, with a nice round head. I should also mention a very special fact about his birth: he was born on 10.10.10. This sure makes his birthday hard to forget for anybody. Yet most people don't believe me that it was a natural and spontaneous birth, not a scheduled one. As if his rare birth date wasn't cool enough all by itself, it turned out to be his father's and also his great grandfather's birthday.

When I was pregnant for a second time, I was told that the doctor who delivered my first boy had already retired. Taking into consideration that his office was an hour drive away from my new home and that obviously he made up a story to use the suction cup to try to enjoy the rest of the Sunday evening, I didn't attempt to verify if he was still available and instead, as is already obvious, chose a different doctor.

Chapter 53: You Are Never Quite Ready for Labor

It's Saturday, and today I reached my milestone and completed 38 weeks of my latest pregnancy. On my last doctor's visit a few days ago, my doctor felt very confident that labor would come spontaneously in the next week or so. I'm about 1.5 cm dilated, and my baby is already positioned very low. I haven't even felt Braxton Hicks contractions yet, so I've been preparing myself psychologically for an induced labor. My close friend in New York has just given birth two weeks ago at 38 weeks after her water broke suddenly in the middle of the night. After hours of intense labor, they had to induce and she ended up having an emergency C-section, as the baby was rather big. Due to the induction, she hemorrhaged heavily for almost 3 days and had to be put on blood transfusion. This news really scared me, but I accepted the fact that if we do have to induce labor, I need to be ready for the possible consequences.

After dinner, my husband and I watch a movie to relax a bit, although I could use some extra sleep. I feel a bit out of place though; I don't quite feel any particular pain, just a bit off. Around midnight, I finally go to bed.

As I'm trying to fall asleep, I feel a sudden wetness. I'm not sure if it's just random discharge, but the idea of my water breaking does cross my mind. Since my water didn't break with my first pregnancy, I'm not quite sure what to look for, whether a puddle of liquid or just a spoonful. It's too late to call anybody, but I send a text message to my friend in New York asking about her experience. Having a newborn, she's probably up all night anyways. She responds right away. Based on her experience, my water did break and will probably continue leaking out in bigger amounts very soon. I also send a text message to my doctor informing him that I might be checking in the hospital in the morning, aware that he isn't in town this weekend. Somehow I think he expected this to happen, probably based on my last check-up. He responds right away, saying that he would prefer I check in the hospital now so his staff can monitor me and give him real-time reports. He's only 2 hours away by car, so if my labor progresses rapidly, he would get on the road right away.

I think I finally realize what's really happening and start freaking out a bit. With my first pregnancy, things were quite different.

Chapter 54: Here Comes Baby no. 2

Yes, my first delivery was very different. This time around, it's about 1 am when I check in at the [same] hospital. By now my contractions are only a minute or two apart, and during the last hour they have intensified tremendously. Around 3 am, I ask for painkillers, as the pain has become quite unbearable, and I have exhausted all my options to control it. The nurse tells me that we have to wait for my doctor to arrive first to assess my condition and approve any painkillers. Time seems to drag endlessly. I eat all my healthy snacks to gain some energy, move as much as I can, work on my breathing, yet I can't wait for it to be over. This time, the pain is much, much stronger than for my first boy.

My doctor arrives around 7 am, all smiley and relaxed, and informs me that everything looks great and we'll be delivering my baby boy very soon. When I desperately ask about painkillers, he nods in agreement, mumbles a name of some medicine we can use and then leaves. What I don't hear is that it's not going to reduce the pain, but will only make me more relaxed and drowsy. I realize that soon after I swallow the pills my nurse gives me. Looking back, it was probably a better option than having an epidural, but at that moment I wanted to kill him.

Although I'm psychologically prepared for any delivery option necessary, in the end I deliver naturally, once again—no suction cup helping me like last time, only lots of pain and even screams at the end, which I never thought could actually come out of me. My boy no. 2 is born at 9:17 am. And just like that, all the pain is gone, and I'm able to breath and smile right away. But I'm sure I'll never do it again. As my grandmother used to say, "One child is too little, and two is too many." We shall see how I handle two boys in my life now.

Chapter 55: Motherhood and Atheism

Growing up in an atheist family, religion was never a part of my life or subject of any interest. Even my religious grandmother was never in favor of the church as an institution, and the only interest I have ever had in churches was its architecture [naturally being an architect].

My husband grew up in an entirely different environment, very religious, but he came out even more non-religious than I did. Naturally, we plan on raising our kids as critical thinkers. But we do face many challenges, such as the school/daycare environment, some friends and my husband's mom, who helps out with the kids every now and then and tries to swing them her way (Catholicism).

So far we are dealing only with our 4.5 year old, who happens to be very attached to his grandma. And since grandma goes to church regularly (almost every day, her busy schedule permitting), her vocabulary and lifestyle fully reflects her dedication to God. When our son was 2 or 3, we had no problem with grandma taking him to church with her every now and then. But now that he's formulating his own opinions and tries to rationalize every new experience, we prefer to keep him away. The fact that he enjoys science and nature helps us out tremendously. We are constantly looking for tools such as books, educational toys or videos that help explaining some of the many questions he's showering us with every day. We realize this is an ongoing challenge, but at the same time all we really want to achieve is to raise free thinkers, so our kids can formulate their own views on God and world creation and are capable of discussing the subject without fear, emotion, and anger.

Chapter 56: Getting Back in Shape After Delivery

Let's be honest, whether due to pregnancy or not, staying in shape after 40 is a job in and of itself. Not only is our metabolism slower now, we might be slowing down overall and become more comfortable with who we are; life gets somewhat settled at a more relaxed pace. Shall I go to the gym today? Nah, I'll go tomorrow. Shall I walk to work or wait for the bus? I'll take a bus since it's Monday. And so on.

Being an athlete all my life, I never thought I would have a problem with weight. Luckily, so far I have not, and I would like it to stay that way. Over the years, I learned a few things about my body that would help me loose unnecessary "love handles" pretty fast, but even these tricks don't work now as they used to. During my first pregnancy, I did yoga stretches and jogged almost daily. But then I didn't have a house and a child; therefore, my time management was much easier. I gained only about 15 pounds during the entire first pregnancy, and after delivery I was back to normal within 2 weeks. Looking back at our first family photo shoot at the beach, I'm quite amazed myself at how things turned out.

I guess I expect it will be similar the second time around. But this time I have a big house, a 4.5-year-old monkey, 3 businesses, and I'm over 40. None of these can stop me, although I gained about 24 pounds total during this pregnancy.

The day of my second child's delivery I'm in a lot of pain and exhausted, so exercising doesn't even cross my mind. The next morning I have to fast and undertake a small surgical procedure of sterilization since my husband and I decided that we are fully satisfied with having 2 children. When I come back to my senses after the surgery, I feel even worse than after the delivery. The third day I have a huge appetite and a need to stretch. But my body isn't ready for anything but rest, and I feel an intense pain immediately after I attempt to do any moves. I do have to take it easy and so I take advantage of being in the hospital to read and rest.

The fourth day I'm released to go home, and although I'm still in pain, I have to get back to my daily routine and end up running around doing errands all day. That definitely doesn't help my recovery, but after a good night's sleep, I'm ready to go back to my morning exercise routine. This consists of a combination of yoga and Pilates stretches with a core and upper body workout. Basically, it's my own version of a full-body workout in 30 minutes. Although I start slow, I feel resistance right away in some parts of my body, mainly in my core (understandably), but also in my overall flexibility. I remind myself of what I went through recently and give myself some time to avoid pain and allow for healing. For instance, I skip my push-up routine for the first few days completely, and only introduce it into my routine a week after delivery. I start with 5 at a time in 2 sets, and after another week I'm back to 10 push-ups in 3 sets. It takes about two weeks to be able to do my full workout without experiencing any pain. I also add core crunches and planks to strengthen my core muscles since I have a little belly left after my pregnancy and unlike the previous time, it isn't disappearing as fast as I was hoping it would.

I'm getting my body back and feel good and strong, but there are still few extra pounds I can't shed. Although everybody is complimenting me on how good I look in such a short time, I don't like the extra handles around my waistline and my butt. It's time to start jogging again.

I realize I haven't been running for about a year now, and although I'm in a decent shape, running does utilize different muscles than yoga or a core workout and I do have a history of bad knees and joint deterioration. Plus, my former running buddy and now a fresh mom warns me that pregnancy can cause loose joints and excessive running can make that condition worse. As Steve Alaniz of Momentum Physical Therapy & Sports Rehab in San Antonio, Texas explains, "*The hormone Relaxin could be a hero and a culprit when it comes to pregnancy. In order to squeeze the watermelon-sized baby through the pelvis, the pelvis needs to widen. Ligaments need to stretch in order to let the pelvis widen. This is all fine and is part of the miracle of life, but Relaxin is non-specific in its targeting of joints to loosen up. It takes effect on all ligaments in the body. This is why many joints feel looser both during and after pregnancy. Relaxin doesn't just disappear once the baby arrives and breastfeeding creates more of the hormone so it may take a while for joints to return to 'normal' after a pregnancy*."

What that all means is that certain types of exercise should be done gradually, maybe even avoided, and additional support of knees and ankles is strongly recommended.

An additional 2 weeks after delivery, I'm running twice a week and monitoring my performance, and I'm happy that I did manage to lose the additional love handles and my weight is now officially back to my pre-pregnancy level at 127 pounds. For the first time in my life, I use a monitoring application on my phone, and my performance is improving each time, even though I don't feel like I'm really pushing myself too much. I'm also making sure my right knee has good support and I'm using gel arch supports in my running shoes, as pregnancy often causes the feet to flatten and can affect overall posture and cause joint problems. My chiropractor also recommends balancing my running with swimming, which I welcome with open arms since swimming is my favorite sport and it's very gentle on the joints. I realize I'm really lucky to have amazing neighbors who allow me to use their 20m-long lap pool anytime I need or fancy my water exercises.

Chapter 57: Depression During Pregnancy and Postpartum

Being pregnant for 9 months, and subsequently caring for a newborn, definitely takes its toll on a woman's body and her mental health. Lasting stress, physical pain, and sleep deprivation can all contribute to a major depressive disorder.

Although I'm not aware of experiencing any depressive states (sometimes you are just too tired and sleepy that you can't feel a thing), I admit there were times both during my pregnancy and after delivery when I was feeling rather "blue" —nothing major I wasn't able to cope with on my own or by talking about it with my close friends, but it wasn't a state of mind I would want to experience again. That just wasn't ME.

As it happens, a new study[29] recently published in the journal JAMA, focuses on this subject and suggests preventive screenings. According to this study

---

[29] Primary Care Screening for and Treatment of Depression in Pregnant and Postpartum Women

of U.S. women evaluated in 2005, 9.1% of pregnant women and 10.2% of postpartum women meet the criteria for a major depressive episode. That's a significant number. Maternal depression can also affect the baby since a mother suffering from depression tends to be less interactive, which can lead to higher rates of emotional and behavioral problems in babies, worse social competence with their peers, and poorer adjustment to the school environment. As the study authors conclude, "*Direct and indirect evidence suggested that screening pregnant and postpartum women for depression may reduce depressive symptoms in women with depression and reduce the prevalence of depression in a given population. Evidence for pregnant women was sparser but was consistent with the evidence for postpartum women regarding the benefits of screening, the benefits of treatment, and screening instrument accuracy.*"

This is where a woman's partner can play a significant role, as he/she might be able to recognize signs of the depression early, help her deal with it, and/or support her in getting help professionally.

Another recent study published in the journal *Anesthesia & Analgesia*[30] found a link between an epidural during childbirth and postpartum depression (PPD). And although some of us may guess that the effect of epidural would be negative, the study actually concluded that epidural labor analgesia was associated with a decreased risk of postpartum depression.

While reading the remarkable "encyclopedia of violence", *The Better Angels of our Nature* by Steven Pinker, I came across a reference to PPD in connection with infanticide[31]. Pinker refers to research by Daly and Wilson and anthropologist Edward Hagen. All of their work suggests that PPD is actually not caused by hormonal malfunctions (there is only a slight link to a measured hormonal imbalance), as PPD is often treated. However, PPD is a result of the mother's emotional struggle on whether to keep her newborn

---

[30] Epidural Labor Analgesia Is Associated with a Decreased Risk of Postpartum Depression: A Prospective Cohort Study

[31] Infanticide (or infant homicide) is the intentional killing of infants or children. Parental infanticide researchers have found that mothers are far more likely than fathers to be the perpetrator for neonaticide (intentional killing during the first 24 hours of life) and slightly more likely to commit infanticide in general.

child or not.

In his 1999 paper called *The Functions of Postpartum Depression*[32], the anthropologist Edward H. Hagen notes: "Numerous studies support the correlation between PPD and lack of social support or indicators of possible infant health and development problems. PPD may be an adaptation that informs mothers that they are suffering or have suffered a fitness cost, that motivates them to reduce or eliminate investment in offspring under certain circumstances, and that may help them negotiate greater levels of investment from others. PPD also appears to be a good model for depression in general."

In their numerous papers on the PPD subject including *The Darwinian Psychology of Discriminative Parental Solicitude*[33] (1988) authors Daly and Wilson suggest that PPD may be a functional component of human parental decision-making instead of a sign of an abnormal psychological state.

---

32 The Functions of Postpartum Depression

33 The Darwinian Psychology of Discriminative Parental Solicitude

I personally find that fascinating. If we look at natural selection as described by Charles Darwin, it's the key mechanism of evolution, for species to survive, and adapt to current conditions. Although we, rational beings, might find selective reproduction cruel, in the animal world, we can observe this phenomenon everywhere.

Chapter 58: Adoption as an Option

As we say in Czech, "Marriage without kids is like a day without sunshine."

Although I always hoped I'd be able to have biological children, one can never tell. Also, women are just half of the equation. Many men these days have problems with fertility for various reasons, including stress, diet, environmental factors, and others. As a result, some couples are unable to have biological children together, which means either using another man's sperm or opting for adoption.

However, being able to "produce" a child naturally is just part of the job. Another part, and much more challenging and demanding, is to raise a child. And raising a child, not just giving a birth is, in my opinion, what makes a true parent. It breaks my heart hearing or reading about cases when biological parents abuse, torture, and even kill their own baby or child, simply because they can't handle the task of parenting, while so many couples that can't have their own children are willing to adopt and would make excellent parents. In some European countries, there are even “drop boxes” installed in many hospitals, where a new mom or a parent can literally drop their baby off anonymously, knowing that their baby will be taken care of and offered for adoption to responsible and loving parents.

An adopted child is not any less your own child. Once you decide to be a parent, all of your children, regardless of their origin, should be measured and loved equally.

Chapter 59: Surrogacy as an Option

As we say in Czech, "An apple does not fall far from the tree."

The options for women who may struggle with infertility or other challenges that keep them from bearing children vary widely. One such option that is becoming increasingly more common is surrogacy. Funny enough, I first learned about surrogacy from an article about the comedian Jimmy Fallon. He and his wife struggled with fertility for about 5 years until they finally considered using a surrogate. Now they have two healthy children, both born via surrogate.

According to data from the American Society for Reproductive Medicine, births via gestational surrogacy have been increasing steadily since 2004. Their latest data indicate that in 2011 there were 1,593 babies born via gestational surrogacy compared to 738 babies seven years earlier in 2004. Very little data is currently being collected about it, but by some estimates, up to 3,000 babies a year are born via surrogacy today.

So what is “surrogacy”, exactly?

Surrogacy is an agreement to carry a pregnancy for intended parents. Going back as far as ancient Mesopotamia (cca 1754 BC), the Babylonian law allowed infertile woman to have another woman bear a child for her and her husband to raise. This practice usually involved the husband as the genetic father and the surrogate as the genetic mother. This form of surrogacy is nowadays considered as ancient, and is no longer practiced. Unlike adoption, when the adopted child might be biologically unrelated to the adopting parents, surrogacy often involves one or both parent’s genetic material. There are cases, however, where the child is born of genetic material from both sides.

Nowadays, there are two main types of surrogacy: gestational and traditional surrogacy.

Gestational surrogacy, also known as host or full surrogacy, means that the surrogate carries a child genetically unrelated to her. The pregnancy results from the transfer of an embryo created by IVF. The embryo can be created using intended father's sperm and intended mother's eggs. Or the embryo can be created using one of the intended parent’s own egg/sperm and the other egg/sperm of a donor, or use both sperm and egg from a donor or a use a donor embryo.

Intended parents may seek a surrogacy arrangement with or without monetary compensation. If the surrogate receives money for the surrogacy arrangement, it is considered commercial surrogacy; if she receives no compensation beyond reimbursement of medical and other reasonable expenses, it is considered altruistic surrogacy.

Cost

In general, the cost for commercial gestational surrogacy ranges from around $70,000 to $200,000 or even beyond, depending on the selected program and state/country of the arrangement. Standard programs vary in the source of the egg donation, IVF insurance coverage, legal needs and other circumstances.

To give an example[34]: if you are using your own eggs to create an embryo, the approximate cost breakdown for US residents could be the following:

---

[34] Source: Circle Surrogacy

Gestational Carrier Related Professional Fees	$22,000.00
Gestational Carrier Related Legal Fees, Expenses and Finalization of Parental Rights	$13,450.00
Gestational Carrier Compensation and Other Expenses	$35,250.00
Licensed Clinical Social Worker Support Fees	$3,500.00
Screening and Background Checks for Carriers and Intended Parents	$1,900.00
TOTAL excluding IVF, insurance, travel, and incidentals	$76,100.00

Traditional surrogacy involves naturally or artificially inseminating a surrogate with intended father's sperm via Intrauterine insemination (IUI), IVF or home insemination. With this method, the resulting child is genetically related to the intended father as well as to the surrogate.

The surrogate can also be artificially inseminated with donor sperm using Intracervical insemination (ICI), IUI or IVF, in which case the resulting child is genetically unrelated to the intended parents but is genetically related to the surrogate. Furthermore, in many jurisdictions the intended parents will need to go through an adoption process to obtain legal rights over the resulting child.

Traditional surrogacy has become very rare these days. Most reputable clinics will work only with the parents' genetic material and/or donor genetic material.

To my huge surprise, most European countries including France, Germany, Italy, Norway, Spain, banned any form of surrogacy. Only a handful of countries around the world allow both commercial and altruistic forms. In the United States, some states allow altruistic surrogacy only, some allow surrogacy for heterosexual married couples only, and others allow only non-commercial surrogacy arrangements. However, most states including Alaska, California, Connecticut, Colorado, Delaware, Florida, Hawaii, allow commercial surrogacy as well. In contrast, states such as Michigan forbid surrogacy by law, and individuals who enter into surrogacy arrangements may be fined up to $50,000 and imprisoned for up to five years. Even liberal states such as New York are strictly against any form of surrogacy, and those who facilitate surrogacy arrangements, such as lawyers and agencies, can be fined in the first instance, and are considered guilty of a felony for the second offense.

When discussing the subject with a close friend, as a possible option if things didn't go well naturally for my husband and me, she referred me to a mutual friend who was a surrogate for a couple in Colorado just a few years back. She carried and gave birth to twins for them, and remained in a close relationship with them since. Also another friend in New York, who couldn't carry on a pregnancy herself due to a genetic predisposition used a surrogate, who successfully carried their twins. I asked both of my friends to give me their side of the story to share with my audience, since each of them experienced surrogacy from a different side.

Liz's story in her own words

"Just as different stories bring intended parents to the decision that surrogacy is their path to having children, surrogates enter the journey with their own backgrounds, experiences, and personal connections to pregnancy and fertility. My husband and I resolved long ago that my own two children were the only babies we would be bringing home. I was fortunate to have very uneventful pregnancies and deliveries, fulfilling my desire to experience natural childbirth with both children. Contrary to some other experiences, I thoroughly enjoyed both pregnancies and births. I knew that perhaps it was something I could offer to others.

Working with a respected surrogacy agency, the journey was relatively seamless. It can, at times, feel more formal than emotional when you have to negotiate with lawyers, take psychological exams, and make sure everyone involved is aware of your menstrual cycle, but it also makes it feel like a transparent process where both parties are involved in how things move forward.

The process of matching a surrogate to intended parents has been described as a cross between a first date and a job interview, which I find very fitting. In our case, we had never met before and had one hour to go from very superficial conversations about our jobs and backgrounds, to philosophical discussions about how many embryos each party is comfortable transferring, or in which cases might each party consider terminating or reducing the number of fetuses. After that short time, you're asked to decide if you want to forever be part of each other's lives. We were fortunate to meet parents who we knew were similar to us in many ways and whose story was important to us.

As with my own pregnancies, everything went according to plan. Nearly all surrogates I have met decide to go down that path because they look fondly on their own pregnancies. This, however, is no guarantee that a surrogate pregnancy will be so easy on your body. While we experienced a textbook transfer, and subsequent twin pregnancy, some women find the surrogate pregnancy to be even more challenging than their own. All agree, however, that once the journey ends, the moments of watching parents hold their babies for the first time make any challenges fly quickly out the window.

The twins' parents live nearby and were able to attend most of the monthly and, eventually weekly, appointments. They took time to get to know our own children and we quickly learned that we had even more in common than we could have realized in our short match meeting. When the time came - at 38 and a half weeks - to deliver the babies, they were both breech and we were facing a C-section. The hospital allowed both my husband and the mother into the operating room. It was a surreal experience, especially since I had never even had an Epidural with my own children. There were at least a dozen people in the room and everything happened quickly. It's hard to recall all of the details of the delivery, but I will not forget watching their mother hold her babies for the first time, after having waited so patiently to be that close to them.

My own children, who were 4 and 5 at the time, found the process fascinating, even assigning nicknames for the babies before they were born. They never questioned why I would do this, or who would be taking the babies home. It reminded me that our children are constantly shaping their world view. What they experience develops their sense of how things operate in the world. While adults have a hard time understanding why someone would choose to do that, or may think it unusual, my children saw it as simply another way that families come together. This may have been one of the most valuable things that our family took from the experience.

Carrying a child for someone else brings a roller coaster of emotion. You feel protective over the lives that have been entrusted to you, equally protective of yourself and your family in the physical and emotional journey you are on, anxious about doing something wrong, annoyed at some of the questions it stirs up with strangers, and thrilled about being part of such a journey. The support network I developed with other surrogates quickly became my rock and my inspiration. There are not many people who can identify with the frank conversations about which injections of hormones you take and where, or why people can't understand that you're not "giving up" a baby.

Getting to know these women is a constant reminder that we each have our stories. Some have gone on to carry for other families, or for the same parents another time. Others have tried, but have struggled to carry a second time. As for me, complications after delivery made for a difficult recovery and I likely would not be able to carry again. This has never been a disappointment, however. Just as I knew I would not carry any more of my own children, I am perfectly content having brought two healthy boys into the world for a loving family. The experience forever impacted who I am and the ways I view starting families. In short, any path is the right path and our own journeys as parents or our role as support systems can sometimes help others find their way."

Limor's story in her own words

"Our twin girls are almost 12 years old now, so our experience goes back about 13 years. We were referred to an attorney, who went through the process of surrogacy with her children herself, and then shifted her practice to help other couples with surrogacy. She hand picked a few possible candidates for us. We lived in New York, and this state does not allow surrogacy by law, at least not the commercial type, which was our case. Therefore, we knew our surrogate would have to be from other states that do allow this kind of arrangement, such as Connecticut. When we met with our first candidate, we felt an instant bond and a sense of comfort. She was a single mom with a 6-year old daughter at that time. We were quite fortunate to find a match right away, since that doesn't always happen.

We went through the process, both legal, and the actual implantation of an embryo, using our own eggs and sperm. It worked on the first try, and we made sure we were involved in the pregnancy as much as we could. We visited her about every month throughout the pregnancy and about every week towards the delivery date.

We both attended the delivery, which was an incredible experience for us. If I was delivering the babies, I would have never been able to see it from this perspective, of course. And since I didn't have the physical discomfort and pain after delivery, I was fresh and ready to care for our newborns day and night. And I sure did enjoy it to the max. Our surrogate became part of the family, we are still very much in touch, and her daughter is about to start college in New York, so she can be even closer to our twins now.

I would definitely recommend using an agency, which specializes on surrogacy, or an attorney, such as ours. I recall us dealing with issues such as having my name being listed on the birth certificate as the "mother", and not the name of our surrogate. The legal aspects of commercial surrogacy can be quite overwhelming and complicated, so professional assistance makes a huge difference."

Chapter 60: The Zika Virus and Pregnancy

As we say in Czech,
"There's no smoke without fire."

Chances are, by the time you are reading this chapter, you are most likely aware of the existence of Zika virus, since media as well as health agencies have been very proactive in educating public about its potential risks. Since research is ongoing in real time, and new (and sometimes conflicting) findings are being regularly announced, the information provided in this chapter is based on findings as of December 8th, 2016.

To date, research has shown that Zika (a flavivirus) is spread primarily by the bite of an infected mosquito of the *Aedes* species, mainly *Aedes aegypti* and *Aedes albopictus*. Both of these species are active during the day as well as night. However, the virus has been found to be transmittable by sexual means as well.

According to CDC data, a total of nearly 4,000 cases of Zika infection have been reported in the United States alone. While most of these cases are travel-related, more than 100 reported cases have originated within the United States. Around the world, more than 60 countries have reported mosquito-borne transmission of the Zika virus.

Women, who are pregnant, might be the most vulnerable to the effects of the virus, since it can cause a birth defect of the brain called *microcephaly*[35] and other severe fetal brain defects. Other complications including defects of the eye, hearing deficits, and impaired growth, have also been detected among fetuses and infants infected with Zika virus in vitro.

Although, currently the most affected areas are those with occurrence of the *Aedes* species, prevention and protection is a key for any woman who is either pregnant or planning on becoming pregnant.

So what does that mean in a practical sense?

---

[35] Microcephaly is a condition where a baby's head is much smaller than expected. During pregnancy, a baby's head grows because the baby's brain grows. Microcephaly can occur because a baby's brain has not developed properly during pregnancy or has stopped growing after birth, which results in a smaller head size. Microcephaly can be an isolated condition, meaning that it can occur with no other major birth defects, or it can occur in combination with other major birth defects.

1. If you are planning on becoming pregnant in the next 6 months or so:

- both you and your partner should avoid traveling to areas most affected by the virus (see current map[36])

- if you do have to travel to areas affected by the virus, protect yourself from any mosquito bites, and have yourself tested upon return and consult your health professional.

2. If you are already pregnant:

- avoid traveling to areas most affected by the virus, and protect yourself from any mosquito bites even in your current home.

- if your partner has to travel to areas affected by the virus, he should get tested upon return and consult his health professional. You should practice protected sex after his return, even if he has tested negative.

Just like with any other infectious disease, prevention is most desirable. However, contracting the Zika virus while you are pregnant, doesn't mean you or

[36] CDC-map of Zika-active countries

your child will suffer any consequences. According to an analysis published in May 2016 in the *New England Journal of Medicine, a* pregnant woman infected with Zika during the first trimester has a probability of 1-13 % of having a child with microcephaly. Other research[37] found that most women infected in their second and third trimesters, had children with no birth defects. However, according to *Morbidity and Mortality Weekly Report*[38] published on December 2, 2016, a study of 13 babies in Brazil infected with Zika in vitro but born without signs of microcephaly found, that 11 of these babies have developed the condition as they have grown older, at 11 or 12 months of age. This finding is definitely very concerning, but again, it doesn't mean that a pregnant woman infected with Zika will give birth to a child who will have any health complications.

Coincidentally, a good friend of mine, who is expecting her first child at 41, was diagnosed with Zika during the first trimester. She has been monitored during the entire pregnancy, is about to give birth, and

---

[37] Zika and the Risk of Microcephaly

[38] Description of 13 Infants Born During October 2015–January 2016 With Congenital Zika Virus Infection Without Microcephaly at Birth in Brazil

the baby has not shown any signs of abnormal growth or concerns for birth defects.

As research continues tirelessly, a prospect for an effective Zika vaccine casts some light on the issue. Although still in preclinical phase, a new DNA-based vaccine has generated a robust and protective antigen-specific antibody and T cell immune responses in animal models. As researchers from The Wistar Institute explain, 100% of the animal models were protected from Zika after vaccination followed by a challenge with the Zika virus. In addition, they were protected from degeneration in the cerebral cortex and hippocampal areas of the brain, while the other cohort showed degeneration of the brain after Zika infection. The lead researcher David B. Weiner, Ph.D., Executive Vice President and Director of the Vaccine Center at The Wistar Institute and the W.W. Smith Charitable Trust Professor in Cancer Research at Wistar, added: "As the threat of Zika continues, these results provide insight into a new aspect of the possibly protective ability of such a vaccine as a preventative approach for Zika infection." The study[39] was published in Nature Research Journal in November 2016.

---

[39] In vivo protection against ZIKV infection and pathogenesis through passive antibody transfer and active immunisation with a prMEnv DNA vaccine

Chapter 61: The Beauty of Parenting

As we say in Czech, "Patience brings roses."

As I'm following my toddler's footsteps in the sand, seconds before the ocean waves wash them off I realize how short and fragile life is. One day you are looking at baby footprints, the next day they are all grown up. And although I feel like I'm having a rough parenting day, questioning some of my decisions, I want to enjoy all these special moments while they last.

Looking back, I never really thought I would become a parent one day; and here I am with two little monkeys on my back. Life has definitely changed. However despite the lack of sleep, lack of "me" time, and body leftovers from both pregnancies, I wouldn't change a thing. Off course I bitch and complain every now and then, just like probably the majority of moms out there do. But then I take pleasure in all the other moments. I enjoy teaching them the good values and skills I have acquired from my own parents, grandparents, my teachers and mentors, as well as my own life lessons.

Patience does bring roses and there are moments when all the hardship and sacrifice melts away instantly and is replaced with pure joy. For the last few years, my now six-year-old son has been surprising me in unexpected moments with statements like: "I love you mommy, you are the best mom in the whole wide world. For real!" Yes, sometimes he uses it as a little emotional blackmail to make up for something I reprimanded him for, but most of the time it comes out of a blue, when we are simply hanging out, or he comes over just to share his love while I'm working. When that happens, it's like time stops for an instant and we are in this happy bubble together. Some parents call it unconditional love, some child's innocence, some call it luck.

As one Chinese proverb says: " To understand your parent's love, you must raise children yourself."

For me, the most important thing I have learned from being a parent, was getting to know myself. Raising my children feels like constantly looking in a mirror, a mirror of time, reflecting on my own mistakes I did as a daughter while growing up, trying to make sense of old situations when my parents acted the way they did, and what that teaches me about my own actions towards my children. It's an ongoing process, and I'm discovering new things every day. Browsing through my own baby album, I realize how familiar those facial grimaces and random action shots of me as a baby appear; as if I was looking at my own children in real time.

In the end, the circle of life must continue no matter what our ideals or beliefs about the future are. And our children will derive a self from who we are, so we-parents-should be the people who we want our children to be. That's the one lesson I have to remind myself every time I'm ready to explode or say something I would probably regret the instant it leaves my lips. Observing my younger son learning from the actions of my older son, is the best reminder of that.

If you made it all the way to this point, I want to thank you for your time. I hope you found a thing or two in this book useful or at least entertaining. If you are planning to become pregnant and are at a similar stage in your life, I wish you the best of luck. From my own experience: patience, persistence and good humor are important components of the process. Along with a good partner and supportive friends, of course.

A Parents' Guide to Children's Vaccinations

By Robert Rivera PhD, 2013

When it comes to vaccinating children, often there is a lot of conflicting information, especially for green parents. One side states that we are better off vaccinating our kids. The other side states that vaccinating our child is wrong and unnecessary. More and more parents are deciding either not to vaccinate their child, or to delay the immunization shots. So what should parents do about vaccination? I thought it would be useful to write on this very important topic on what to look for when deciding on whether to vaccinate your child.

Very few things in life are guaranteed. Driving a car carries risk. So does walking on a sidewalk. Every day we make decisions by asking ourselves: will the benefits of our decision outweigh the risks? When it comes to vaccinating our child, the thought process is no different. We provide an objective perspective of all the important aspects that one must consider when doing your own vaccine benefit risk evaluation.

Let's get started with the benefits of vaccination!

Benefits of vaccines

Although the history of vaccines dates back to the 18th century, it was around the beginning of the 20th century when scientists started using vaccines to prevent rabies, rubella, measles, diphtheria, and polio among many others. Vaccines have dramatically reduced (and in some cases eradicated) many serious diseases. For thousands of years, the life expectancy of human beings hovered around 30 years or so. Only at the beginning of the 20th century was there a dramatic change. Many health experts attribute two main factors to the radical increase in life expectancy: antibiotics and vaccines. Among scientists there's virtually no debate about vaccines being able to immunize people against diseases. For some perspective, we provide some statistics:

• ***Diphtheria*** cases peaked in 1921 at over 200,000 in the United States. That same year, William Park ran a program to compare diphtheria cases among vaccinated children and those that were not vaccinated. The program included 180,000 children. He found that untested and unvaccinated children were 4 times more likely to suffer from the disease than vaccinated children[40]. In 1997, there were only 5 cases of diphtheria[41].

• About 500,000 cases of ***measles*** occurred each year in the United States until 1963. That same year the first measles vaccine was licensed. When an outbreak of measles hit the U.S. in 1989, it affected mostly areas with low vaccination rates[42]. In 1999, there were only 86 cases of the disease[43].

• ***Measles*** killed over 500,000 children around the world in 2003, with the highest death toll occurring in Africa. People in the U.S. who have not been vaccinated against measles are 35 times more likely to contract the disease than vaccinated ones[44].

---

[40] The History of Vaccines

[41] Risk, A practical guide for deciding what's really safe and what's really dangerous in the world around you

[42] The History of Vaccines -measles

[43] Risk, A practical guide for deciding what's really safe and what's really dangerous in the world around you

[44] Health Consequences of Religious and Philosophical Exemptions From Immunization Laws: Individual and Societal Risk of Measles

• ***Pertussis*** (also known as whooping cough) kills about 300,000 children a year around the world[45].

• ***Influenza type b*** (Haemophilus influenzae or Hib) affected 1 in 200 children just before the vaccine was introduced in 1988. Hib was the leading cause of bacterial meningitis. Between 15 and 30% of affected children became hearing impaired, and approximately 420 children died every year despite antibiotic therapy. In addition, the Hib vaccine has prevented the leading cause of acquired mental retardation in the U.S. By 1998, vaccination of pre-school children reduced the number of Hib cases by more than 99%[46].

• ***Rubella*** is a viral disease that, if it affects a woman in the early stages of pregnancy, can lead to serious birth defects in at least 20% of incidences[47]. During the 1960s many infants were born with deafness, blindness, heart disease, mental retardation, and other birth defects because of Rubella.

Not only do vaccines prevent the development of potentially serious diseases, children vaccination programs help to protect the entire community by

---

[45] Unicef: Immunization: Why are children dying?
[46] Statement on Risk vs Benefit of Vaccinations

[47] CDC-Rubella

reducing the spread of infectious agents[48]. Generally, doctors recommend several vaccines for children, some more optional than others depending on the situation and the country you live in.

Now that we've looked at the benefits of vaccination, it's time to evaluate the risks involved.

Vaccine side effects: myth or fact? Parents' perception

Vaccines do pose some health risks, and that's one of the reasons parents do not feel at ease about vaccination. Mistrust of pharmaceutical companies is another reason parents are hesitant to vaccinate their children, and who can blame them for feeling this way. The increased number of vaccines used on children is also worrisome to parents. However, in a way, some of the controversy surrounding vaccines is due to their early success. Vaccines were so efficient in reducing the prevalence of diseases that the public concern for these diseases diminished, and the fear about their side effects became the focus. If parents can't perceive the benefits of immunization, then they will focus on the things that they can hear, see, and feel. For the most part, many parents go by what they hear. Research has

---

[48] Statement on Risk vs Benefit of Vaccinations

suggested that parents in the United States pay the most attention to what their partner has to say, followed by their pediatrician and friends and family[49]. The findings imply that social networks have a big influence on parents' decision and help in shaping their beliefs in vaccines. It's extremely uncommon to see parents write on social networks, "We are so happy we just vaccinated our child." Instead, many postings on social networks are either about side effects, or about vaccines being unnecessary.

Proven vaccine side effects

For the most part, side effects from vaccines tend to be mild: redness, pain, congestion, runny nose, and low fever. For the majority of vaccines, severe allergic reactions are the worst possible side effect; although pneumonia (varicella vaccine), prolonged muscle pain (tetanus and diphtheria vaccine) and more serious issues are also possible. Severe side effects are mainly very rare, with a 1 in a million chance or so. For comparison, TVs injure slightly over 2 in 10,000 children

---

[49] The Impact of Social Networks on Parents' Vaccination Decisions

in the U.S.[50] The CDC has information on verified vaccine side effects[51] and reported side effects that are not yet scientifically proven to be caused by vaccines[52]. The CDC together with the U.S. Food and Drug Administration (FDA) has several tools in place to ensure the risk of the use of vaccines is minimized. A very useful one is the Vaccine Adverse Event Reporting System (VAERS), which lets you report and access side effects of using vaccines[53]. They use this data to actively monitor the performance of vaccines. Tips for a less stressful vaccine experience are also provided[54]. Finally, the Health Resources and Services Administration agency provides a table with time periods for side effects to occur (if any) for many vaccines[55]. Parents should be aware that there are a lot of side effects claims spreading through social networks

---

[50] Television-Related Injuries to Children in the United States

[51] CDC: Facts for Parents: Diseases & the Vaccines that Prevent Them

[52] CDC: Possible Side-effects from Vaccines

[53] The Vaccine Adverse Event Reporting System

[54] CDC: For Parents: Vaccines for Your Children

[55] U.S. Department of Health and Human Services: Vaccine Compensation

and websites that are simply incorrect or based on misinterpretations of facts. We will discuss some of these shortly.

Any vaccines that don't work or have too many side effects?

For most vaccines, currently the pros outweigh the cons, but there is some debate among the experts over certain vaccines.

In 1976, there was a swine flu outbreak in Fort Dix, New Jersey. It prompted a mass immunization program. It was later determined that although with a 1 in a million chance, the swine flu vaccine might cause Guillain-Barré syndrome[56], a disorder affecting the peripheral nervous system. Given that the swine flu outbreak was relatively not harmful and the potential serious side effect of the vaccine, the incident had a wide societal and political impact.

More recently, Gardasil, an HPV vaccine available since 2006 has had its share of controversy.

---

[56] Vaccines and Guillain-Barré syndrome

Among the arguments fueling the debate are[57]:

- The amount of years of immunization that the vaccine provides is unknown,
- It only protects against four strains of HPV
- Women must understand that pap smears are still needed,
- More research is needed to have a better understanding of its side effects[58].

Despite the fact that most vaccines currently have more benefits than risks, new vaccines, changes in formulations, and procedures happen all the time, so it's wise to stay on top of the latest news.

False claims related to the use of vaccines

Vaccines cause autism:

- Jenny McCarthy and Jim Carrey are two celebrities who argue vehemently against vaccines and claim links to autism. McCarthy has even written a few books on the subject.

---

[57] National Cancer Institute, Human Papillomavirus (HPV) Vaccines

[58] Gardasil HPV Vaccine Safety Assessed In Most Comprehensive Study To Date

- In a 1998 press conference, Andrew Wakefield stated that his published scientific paper found a link between the MMR vaccine and the onset of autism. This caused a drop in vaccinations in England and an over 2,400% rise in measles cases between 1998 and 2008. When other scientists couldn't reproduce the results, a necessary step in scientific research, and an investigation was conducted. It was found that Dr. Wakefield had a conflict of interest (for example children were recruited by a lawyer with a lawsuit against vaccine manufacturers) and that his study had other fatal flaws[59]. But the damage caused by the publicity had already been done. To this day we still see many who claim that there is a link between autism and the use of the MMR or other vaccines.

- Many of the watchdog agencies do take the public concerns seriously and in 1999, *thimerosal*, a mercury containing preservative found in some vaccines, was reduced or eliminated as a precaution, although scientific evidence did not show a link between thimerosal exposure and autism[60]. It should be

[59] Lancet retracts Wakefield's MMR paper

[60] CDC: Do vaccines cause autism spectrum disorder?

noted that a change in thimerosal content did not reduce the autism rates in the U.S.

Many of the diseases are no longer epidemics, so the corresponding vaccines are unnecessary

- Since many of these diseases are no longer epidemics in the United States, some parents incorrectly assume that the risk of contracting the disease is lower than the risk of their child experiencing an adverse reaction to the vaccine. However, many of these diseases are still common in other countries. For example, the mumps outbreak that occurred in the U.S. in 2006 was probably introduced from an epidemic in Great Britain[61]. Outbreaks of measles and whooping cough have occurred in recent years across the U.S. including the recent so-called Disney linked measles outbreak in 2014.

Whooping cough vaccines are making children more likely to suffer from the disease

---

[61] Immunizations for Public Health: Mumps

- The incidence of the disease has increased in recent years, but there is no evidence to support that vaccines are at fault. This myth might have resulted from misinterpretation of results from recent research. The truth is that children who do not take the pertussis vaccine are at least 8 times more likely to suffer from the disease[62] (one study argues 23 times[63]).

- The case numbers of many diseases started decreasing before the introduction of vaccines—Historical data shows this claim to be false. Even when considering better sanitation and medical service systems, vaccination has been found to play a major role in the reduction of infectious diseases.

- Vaccines have high levels of aluminum in them—Some vaccines use aluminum to boost the immune response to the vaccine. The levels of aluminum are in fact similar to the amount found in a liter of infant formula[64].

---

[62] CDC: Pertussis (Whooping Cough)

[63] Parental Refusal of Pertussis Vaccination Is Associated With an Increased Risk of Pertussis Infection in Children

[64] The Children's Hospital of Philadelphia: Vaccine Ingredients

- Vaccines cause autism, sudden infant death syndrome, diabetes and other diseases—Recent studies do not support any of these arguments[65].

- Natural methods of enhancing immunity, such as breastfeeding and a healthy diet are enough to prevent diseases[66]. While good nutrition and other healthy actions do indeed lead to a better immune system, it is not enough to protect us from many diseases.

- Doctors, pharmaceuticals, and/or anyone that is for vaccines, says so because they are getting money—This is an unfair statement often made against supporters of vaccines. Ironically, one of the main faces of the anti-vaccine movement, Andrew Wakefield, did have financial interests when he made his claims against vaccines.

- There are simply too many vaccines in the vaccination schedule, increasing the chances of adverse events—Currently, there is no scientific evidence supporting this argument. But this is a valid

---

[65] Childhood Vaccines Cleared of Autism, Diabetes Link in New Report

[66] Immunizations for Public Health (I4PH)

concern for parents. Whenever there is a change in the vaccine schedule, this statement must be reconsidered.

Many links between vaccines and diseases have been claimed, but most of them have been debunked[67]. The American Academy of Pediatrics also provides a list of studies debunking many of the side effects and statements discussed above[68].

Parents do have some very valid concerns about vaccines. However, it's important to avoid making conclusions too hastily. A 1998 study found that Australia, Japan, the Russian Federation, and many European countries experienced pertussis outbreaks after pertussis vaccination programs were suspended due to misinformation. Each country found it crucial to reinstate the pertussis vaccine into the vaccination program[69].

Tips for parents about vaccines:

Take a look at the Vaccine Information

---

[67] Adverse Effects of Vaccines: Evidence and Causality

[68] Vaccine Safety: Examine the Evidence

[69] Statement on Risk vs Benefit of Vaccinations

Statements for each vaccine[70]. They provide information on benefits, risks, and who should avoid each vaccine.

Do some research through the CDC and other watch dogs about the latest vaccines since the formulations and vaccines change routinely.

Check conditions for which a patient shouldn't take a given vaccine and tell your doctor if you have any concerns.

Report to the doctor current illness or medical conditions. Some vaccines are postponed if patients have moderate or severe illness.

Be wary of info available through social media and unestablished websites. A lot of it is incorrect.

After giving a vaccine to your child, look for anything unusual such as fever or unusual behavior. Signs of a serious allergic reaction may include difficulty breathing, wheezing, hives, weakness, dizziness, paleness, or accelerated heart beat. If such signs are present, contact a doctor immediately.

Use the Vaccine Adverse Event Reporting

---

[70] CDC: Vaccine Information Statements (VIS)

System (VAERS) to report or find about the side effects of using vaccines[71].

When informed about a side effect, ask yourself: Does the claimed side effect rely on scientific data? – And someone saying so is not enough. Verify the scientific evidence yourself– not only whether it truly exists, but also whether it is a reputable source (these days, there are even fake scientific journals out there), if it has been independently reproduced and validated, and whether there is agreement among experts.

If you want to do your own research on the topic, try checking what universities have to say about the topic. They often have excellent non-technical information available for the public. For example, in Google, you may type '*children vaccines side effects site:.edu*' (no quotes). Then only university websites will show in your queries.

So do the benefits of vaccinating your child outweigh the risks?

---

[71] The Vaccine Adverse Event Reporting System (VAERS)

For the majority of vaccines available, the answer is a resounding yes. But this is not necessarily true for all vaccines available and all situations. Parents should evaluate the benefits and risks of each vaccine separately, according to the most up-to-date data and each individual scenario. Additionally, it is wise to stay on top of the latest news from the watchdogs.

References

[1] **Parental age and the risk of autism spectrum disorders: findings from a Swedish population-based cohort**; *International Journal of Epidemiology, 2014:*
http://ije.oxfordjournals.org/content/43/1/107

[2] **The parenting of preschool children by older mothers in the United Kingdom;** *European Journal of Developmental Psychology, 2014:*
http://discovery.ucl.ac.uk/1427729/

[3] **The health and development of children born to older mothers in the United Kingdom;** *The BMJ* (formerly the *British Medical Journal*), *2012:*
http://www.bmj.com/content/345/bmj.e5116?variant=abstract

[4] **Women 35 and older are at decreased risk of having anatomically abnormal child,** *Society for Maternal-Fetal Medicine, 2014:*
http://www.smfmnewsroom.org/2014/01/study-

suggests-women-35-and-older-are-at-decreased-risk-of-having-anatomically-abnormal-child/

[5] **Congenital defect or birth defect:** http://www.who.int/mediacentre/factsheets/fs370/en/

[6] **Since we're talking science,** in most countries male births are slightly higher than girl births, Specifically, for each conception there's about a 52% chance it will be a boy.

[7] **Father's diet before conception;** *McGill University, 2013* http://www.sciencedaily.com/releases/2013/12/131210113315.htm

[8] **New blood test for Down's syndrome and other genetic abnormalities:** *Ultrasound in Obstetrics & Gynecology, 2013* http://www.sciencedaily.com/releases/2013/06/130607085203.htm

[9] **How Birth Control Could Affect Your Fertility;** *Parenting Magazine*. http://www.parenting.com/article/how-birth-control-could-affect-your-fertility

[10] **Light drinking during pregnancy is not linked to adverse behavioural or cognitive outcomes in childhood**, *BJOG, 2013*
http://www.bjog.org/details/news/4608611/BJOG_study_Light_drinking_during_pregnancy_is_not_linked_to_adverse_behavioural_.html

[11] **Danish studies suggest low and moderate drinking in early pregnancy has no adverse effects on children aged five;** *BJOG, 2012, Volume 119, Issue 10, pages 1201–1210, September 2012*
http://www.bjog.org/details/news/2085661/Danish_studies_suggest_low_and_moderate_drinking_in_early_pregnancy_has_no_adver.html

[12] **Prenatal exposure to alcohol, and gender differences on child mental health at age seven years,** *Journal of Epidemiology and Community Health, 11. November 2013*
http://jech.bmj.com/content/early/2013/11/11/jech-2013202956.full.pdf?ijkey=c5jz5ccU2lk9MSW&keytype=ref

[13] **HCG or human chorionic gonadotropin, the pregnancy hormone,**

http://americanpregnancy.org/while-pregnant/hcg-levels/

[14] **"IT" referring to dead fetus**

[15] **Omphalocele**
https://en.wikipedia.org/wiki/Omphalocele

[16] **Gastroschisis**
http://www.cdc.gov/ncbddd/birthdefects/gastroschisis.html

[17] **Fetal Omphalocele Detected Early in Pregnancy: Associated Anomalies and Outcomes;** *Journal of the Radiological Society of North America, 2004*
http://pubs.rsna.org/doi/abs/10.1148/radiol.2321030795

[18] **Increasing Prevalence of Gastroschisis-14 States, 1995–2012**; *CDC. 2016*
http://www.cdc.gov/mmwr/volumes/65/wr/mm6502a2.htm?s_cid=mm6502a2_w

[19] **Cell-free DNA Analysis for Noninvasive Examination of Trisomy;** *New England Journal of Medicine, 2015*

http://www.nejm.org/doi/full/10.1056/nejmoa1407349#t
=article

[20] **Prenatal maternal stress: effects on pregnancy and the (unborn) child,** *journal Early Human Development, 2002*
http://www.sciencedirect.com/science/article/pii/S0378
378202000750
Stress during pregnancy is associated with developmental outcome in infancy, *Journal of Child Psychology and Psychiatry, 2003*
http://www.ncbi.nlm.nih.gov/pubmed/12959490
Psychosocial stress in pregnancy and its relation to low birth weight, *BMJ, 1984*
http://www.bmj.com/content/288/6425/1191?variant=a
bstract

[21] **Low-Grade Chronic Inflammation in Pregnant Women With Polycystic Ovary Syndrome: A Prospective Controlled Clinical Study.** *The Journal Of Clinical Endocrinology & Metabolism. 2014*
http://press.endocrine.org/doi/abs/10.1210/jc.2014-
1214

[22] **Inflammation in Pregnancy Strongly Linked to Schizophrenia,** *American Journal of Psychiatry, 2014*

http://www.medscape.com/viewarticle/831135

[23] **Brain's Inflammatory Response in Overdrive May Contribute to Common Brain Disorders,** *Society of Neuroscience, 2014*
http://www.sfn.org/Press-Room/News-Release-Archives/2014/Brains-Inflammatory-Response-in-Overdrive-May-Contribute-to-Common-Brain-Disorders

[24] **I'm Autistic, And Believe Me, It's A Lot Better Than Measles:**
https://medium.com/the-archipelago/im-autistic-and-believe-me-its-a-lot-better-than-measles-78cb039f4bea#.sfijur845

[25] **Immunology 101 Series: To Keep You and Your Baby Safe, Vaccines Are Expected When You're Expecting,** *Colorado Children's Immunalization Coalition*
http://teamvaccine.com/2014/06/12/immunology-101-series-to-keep-you-and-your-baby-safe-vaccines-are-expected-when-youre-expecting/
Vaccines for pregnant women:
http://www.cdc.gov/vaccines/pubs/downloads/f_preg_chart.pdf

[26] **Association Between Obstetric Mode of Delivery and Autism Spectrum Disorder: A Population-Based Sibling Design Study**, *JAMA Psychiatry, 2015*
http://archpsyc.jamanetwork.com/article.aspx?articleid=2323630

[27] **Why Are so Many Kids Allergic to Peanuts,** *Popular Science, 2008*
http://www.popsci.com/scitech/article/2008-12/why-are-so-many-kids-allergic-peanuts
Peanut Allergy Cases Triple in 10 Years, *Live Science, 2010*
http://www.livescience.com/8268-peanut-allergy-cases-triple-10-years.html
FARE (Food Allergy Research & Education)
http://www.foodallergy.org/facts-and-stats

[28] **Children at Lower Risk for Peanut, Tree Nut Allergies if Moms Ate More Nuts While Pregnant,** *JAMA Pediatrics, 2013*
http://media.jamanetwork.com/news-item/children-lower-risk-peanut-tree-nut-allergies-moms-ate-nuts-pregnant/

[29] **Primary Care Screening for and Treatment of Depression in Pregnant and Postpartum Women;**

Evidence Report and Systematic Review for the US Preventive Services Task Force, *JAMA journal, 2016* http://jama.jamanetwork.com/article.aspx?articleid=2484344

[30] **Epidural Labor Analgesia Is Associated with a Decreased Risk of Postpartum Depression: A Prospective Cohort Study;**
journal Anesthesia & Analgesia, August 2014
http://journals.lww.com/anesthesia-analgesia/Fulltext/2014/08000/Epidural_Labor_Analgesia_Is_Associated_with_a.21.aspx

[31] **Infanticide** (or infant homicide) is the intentional killing of infants or children. Parental infanticide researchers have found that mothers are far more likely than fathers to be the perpetrator for neonaticide (intentional killing during the first 24 hours of life) and slightly more likely to commit infanticide in general.

[32] **The Functions of Postpartum Depression,** E. H. Hagen, Department of Anthropology, UCSB, 1999
http://anthro.vancouver.wsu.edu/media/PDF/Hagen_1999_The_functions_of_postpartum_depression.pdf
Postpartum depression as an adaptation to paternal and kin exploitation, E. H. Hagen, 1996.

Reproductive Decision-Making and Postpartum Depression, E. H. Hagen, 1998

[33] **The Darwinian Psychology of Discriminative Parental Solicitude**, M.Daly and M.Wilson, 1988
Discriminative parental solicitude: a biological perspective, M.Daly and M.Wilson
Journal of Marriage and the Family, 1980
Sex, Evolution, and Behavior, M.Daly and M.Wilson
Wadsworth Publishing Company, 1983
A sociobiological analysis of human infanticide. In Infanticide: Comparative and Evolutionary Perspectives, M.Daly and M.Wilson
Aldine, 1984
Discriminative parental solicitude and the relevance of evolutionary models to the analysis of motivational systems, M.Daly and M.Wilson
The MIT Press, 1995

[34] **Circle Surrogacy**
http://www.circlesurrogacy.com/costs

[35] **Microcephaly** is a condition where a baby's head is much smaller than expected. During pregnancy, a baby's head grows because the baby's brain grows. Microcephaly can occur because a baby's brain has not

developed properly during pregnancy or has stopped growing after birth, which results in a smaller head size. Microcephaly can be an isolated condition, meaning that it can occur with no other major birth defects, or it can occur in combination with other major birth defects.

[36] **CDC-map of Zika-active countries**
www.cdc.gov/zika/geo/active-countries

[37] **Zika and the Risk of Microcephaly,** *New England Journal of Medicine, July 2016*
http://www.nejm.org/doi/full/10.1056/NEJMp1605367

[38] **Description of 13 Infants Born During October 2015–January 2016 With Congenital Zika Virus Infection Without Microcephaly at Birth in Brazil,** *CDC, December 2016*
https://www.cdc.gov/mmwr/volumes/65/wr/mm6547e2.htm?s_cid=mm6547e2_w

[39] **In vivo protection against ZIKV infection and pathogenesis through passive antibody transfer and active immunisation with a prMEnv DNA vaccine**
Nature Research Journal, November 2016
http://www.nature.com/articles/npjvaccines201621

[40] **The History of Vaccines**
http://www.historyofvaccines.org/content/timelines/diphtheria

[41] **Risk, A practical guide for deciding what's really safe and what's really dangerous in the world around you,** *David Ropeik and George Gray*

[42] **The History of Vaccines-Measles**
http://www.historyofvaccines.org/content/timelines/measles

[43] **Risk, A practical guide for deciding what's really safe and what's really dangerous in the world around you,** *David Ropeik and George Gray*

[44] **Health Consequences of Religious and Philosophical Exemptions From Immunization Laws: Individual and Societal Risk of Measles**
http://jama.jamanetwork.com/article.aspx?articleid=190649

[45] **Unicef: Immunization: Why are children dying?**
http://www.unicef.org/immunization/index_why.html

[46] **Statement on Risk vs Benefit of Vaccinations by**

David Satcher, M.D., PH.D., *U.S. Department of Health and Human Services*
http://www.hhs.gov/asl/testify/t990803a.html

[47] **CDC-Rubella**
http://www.cdc.gov/rubella/about/index.html

[48] **Statement on Risk vs Benefit of Vaccinations by David Satcher, M.D., PH.D.,** *U.S. Department of Health and Human Services*
http://www.hhs.gov/asl/testify/t990803a.html

[49] **The Impact of Social Networks on Parents' Vaccination Decisions,** *Journal Pediatrics, 2013*
http://pediatrics.aappublications.org/content/early/2013/04/10/peds.2012-2452

[50] **Television-Related Injuries to Children in the United States,** *1990–2011, Journal Pediatrics, 2013*
http://pediatrics.aappublications.org/content/early/2013/07/17/peds.2013-1086.abstract

[51] **CDC: Facts for Parents: Diseases & the Vaccines that Prevent Them**
http://www.cdc.gov/vaccines/vpd-vac/fact-sheet-parents.html

[52] **CDC: Possible Side-effects from Vaccines**
http://www.cdc.gov/vaccines/vac-gen/side-effects.htm#mmr

[53] **The Vaccine Adverse Event Reporting System (VAERS)**
http://vaers.hhs.gov/index

[54] **CDC: For Parents: Vaccines for Your Children**
http://www.cdc.gov/vaccines/parents/tools/tips-factsheet.html

[55] **U.S. Department of Health and Human Services: Vaccine Compensation**
http://www.hrsa.gov/vaccinecompensation/data/

[56] **Vaccines and Guillain-Barré syndrome,** *US National Library of Medicine National Institutes of Health, 2009*
http://www.ncbi.nlm.nih.gov/pubmed/19388722

[57] **National Cancer Institute, Human Papillomavirus (HPV) Vaccines**
http://www.cancer.gov/about-cancer/causes-prevention/risk/infectious-agents/hpv-vaccine-fact-sheet

[58] **Gardasil HPV Vaccine Safety Assessed In Most Comprehensive Study To Date,** *Forbes, 2015*
http://www.forbes.com/sites/tarahaelle/2015/07/15/gardasil-hpv-vaccine-safety-assessed-in-most-comprehensive-study-to-date/#69d0907f53ad

[59] **Lancet retracts Wakefield's MMR paper,** *The BMJ, 2010*
http://www.bmj.com/content/340/bmj.c696

[60] **CDC: Do vaccines cause autism spectrum disorder?**
http://www.cdc.gov/ncbddd/autism/topics.html

[61] **Immunizations for Public Health: Mumps**
http://www.immunizationinfo.org/es/issues/general/vaccine-misinformation

[62] **CDC: Pertussis (Whooping Cough)**
http://www.cdc.gov/pertussis/about/faqs.html

[63] **Parental Refusal of Pertussis Vaccination Is Associated With an Increased Risk of Pertussis Infection in Children,** *Journal Pediatrics, 2009*
http://pediatrics.aappublications.org/content/123/6/1446

[64] **The Children's Hospital of Philadelphia: Vaccine Ingredients**
http://www.chop.edu/service/vaccine-education-center/vaccine-safety/vaccine-ingredients/aluminum.html

[65] **Childhood Vaccines Cleared of Autism, Diabetes Link in New Report,** *Nature Magazine, 2011*
http://www.scientificamerican.com/article.cfm?id=childhood-vaccines-cleared-of-autism-diabetes-link-new-report

[66] **Immunizations for Public Health (I4PH)**
http://www.immunizationinfo.org/

[67] **Adverse Effects of Vaccines: Evidence and Causality,** *The National Academies of Sciences, Engineering, Medicine, 2011*
http://www.iom.edu/Reports/2011/Adverse-Effects-of-Vaccines-Evidence-and-Causality.aspx

[68] **Vaccine Safety: Examine the Evidence,** *American Academy of Pediatrics, 2013*
https://www.aap.org/en-us/Documents/immunization_vaccine_studies.pdf

[69] **Statement on Risk vs Benefit of Vaccinations by David Satcher, M.D., PH.D.,** *U.S. Department of Health and Human Services*
http://www.hhs.gov/asl/testify/t990803a.html

[70] **CDC: Vaccine Information Statements (VIS)**
http://www.cdc.gov/vaccines/hcp/vis/index.html

[71] **The Vaccine Adverse Event Reporting System (VAERS)**
https://vaers.hhs.gov/index

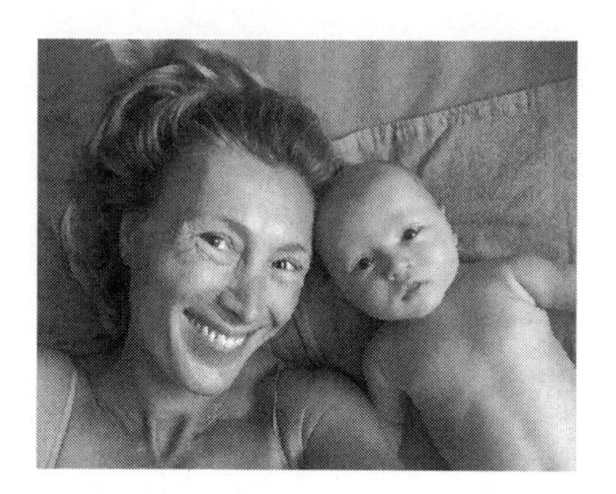

Katka Konecna-Rivera is an architect focused on sustainable design as well as a filmmaker, writer, personal wellness coach, co-founder of Living Green with Baby, and mom to Luca, age 6 years and tot Kai. Katka lives with her family in Puerto Rico and also divides her time between New York and Prague.

Born and raised in Prague, Czech Republic, Katka performed in theater since age seven. Her fascination for arts led her to attend School of Fine Arts, where she mastered everything from classical charcoal drawing to oil painting and metal sculpture. Later, she went on to study engineering to have an understanding of the technical background and principles for her creations, followed by studies in architecture at Czech Technical University. She spent two years gaining practical experiences in the United States and as a guest student at Harvard and Southern California Institute of Architecture. Upon returning to Prague, she took film studies at Academy of Performing Arts while completing her degree in architecture. After graduation she moved to New York City to practice architecture and launched her own furniture collection. She studied dramatic writing at New York University and it was here--with all her experience to bear--that she began writing, producing, and directing her own films. While expecting her first baby, she co-founded Living Green with Baby, which also inspired her book writing. The Art of Pregnancy After 40 is her first published book from The Simple Green Life Book Series.

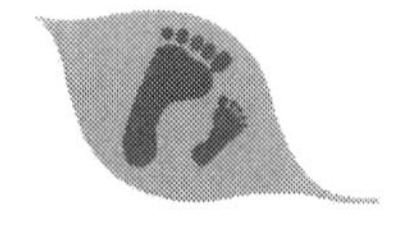

Made in the USA
Middletown, DE
15 January 2018